CAREGIVING

BIBLICAL INSIGHTS FROM A CAREGIVER'S JOURNEY

JIMMIE AARON KEPLER

POETRY AND PRAYER PRESS

CONTENTS

INTRODUCTION	1
CHAPTER 1 *What's With The Bloody Spot?*	3
1.1 My Story	3
1.2 It's Okay to be Afraid	7
1.3 Bible Verse	7
1.4 What the Verse Means	7
1.5 Pray Using Scripture	8
1.6 Responding to God's Hope	9
1.7 Takeaway	9
CHAPTER 2 *How to be Courageous*	11
2.1 My Story	11
2.2 How to Be Courageous	12
2.3 Bible Verse	12
2.4 What the Verse Means	13
2.5 Pray Using Scripture	13
2.6 Responding to God's Hope	13
2.7 Takeaway	14
CHAPTER 3 *You Have Permission to Cry*	15
3.1 My Story	15
3.2 Tears are Normal	16
3.3 Bible Verse	16
3.4 What the Verses Mean	16
3.5 Pray Using Scripture	17
3.6 Responding to God's Hope	17
3.7 Takeaway	18

CHAPTER 4 — 19
How to Rest in God

- 4.1 My Story — 19
- 4.2 Resting in the Lord — 20
- 4.3 Bible Verse — 21
- 4.4 What the Verse Means — 21
- 4.5 Pray Using Scripture — 21
- 4.6 Responding to God's Hope — 21
- 4.7 Takeaway — 22

CHAPTER 5 — 23
How to Have Real Deliverance

- 5.1 My Story — 23
- 5.2 Deliverance for the Believer is in Jesus Christ — 24
- 5.3 Bible Verse — 25
- 5.4 What the Verse Means — 25
- 5.5 Pray Using Scripture — 25
- 5.6 Responding to God's Hope — 26
- 5.7 Takeaway — 26

CHAPTER 6 — 27
Any Delay Could Be Life Threatening

- 6.1 My Story — 27
- 6.2 Hearing God's Voice — 29
- 6.3 Bible Verse — 29
- 6.4 What the Verse Means — 29
- 6.5 Pray Using Scripture — 30
- 6.6 Responding to God's Hope — 30
- 6.7 Takeaway — 30

CHAPTER 7 — 31
The Therapeutic Value of Romantic Comedies

- 7.1 My Story — 31
- 7.2 Learning to Laugh — 33
- 7.3 Bible Verse — 33
- 7.4 What the Verse Means — 33
- 7.5 Pray Using Scripture — 33
- 7.6 Responding to God's Hope — 33
- 7.7 Takeaway — 34

CHAPTER 8 — 35
How to Use Your Remaining Time

- 8.1 My Story — 35
- 8.2 Use the Time God Has Given You — 36
- 8.3 Bible Verse — 37
- 8.4 What the Verse Means — 37
- 8.5 Pray Using Scripture — 37
- 8.6 Responding to God's Hope — 37
- 8.7 Takeaway — 38

CHAPTER 9 — 39
The Source of Real Peace

- 9.1 My Story — 39
- 9.2 Real Peace Comes from God — 41
- 9.3 Bible Verse — 41
- 9.4 What the Verse Means — 41
- 9.5 Prayer Using Scripture — 42
- 9.6 Responding to God's Hope — 42
- 9.7 Takeaway — 42

CHAPTER 10 — 43
How to Have Real Direction For Your Life

- 10.1 My Story — 43
- 10.2 Thy Word — 44
- 10.3 Bible Verse — 44
- 10.4 What the Verse Means — 44
- 10.5 Pray Using Scripture — 45
- 10.6 Responding to God's Hope — 45
- 10.7 Takeaway — 45

CHAPTER 11 — 47
How to Trust God

- 11.1 My Story — 47
- 11.2 Trusting God — 49
- 11.3 Bible Verse — 49
- 11.4 What the Verse Means — 49
- 11.5 Pray Using Scripture — 50
- 11.6 Responding to God's Hope — 50
- 11.7 Takeaway — 50

CHAPTER 12 — 51
How to Have Real Prosperity

12.1 My Story — 51
12.2 Real Prosperity is in the Lord Jesus Christ — 52
12.3 Bible Verse — 52
12.4 What the Verse Means — 52
12.5 Pray Using Scripture — 53
12.6 Responding to God's Hope — 53
12.7 Takeaway — 53

CHAPTER 13 — 55
Do Not Lose Heart

13.1 My Story — 55
13.2 Not Losing Heart — 56
13.3 Bible Verse — 56
13.4 What the Verse Means — 57
13.5 Pray Using Scripture — 57
13.6 Responding to God's Hope — 57
13.7 Takeaway — 58

CHAPTER 14 — 59
Where to Look When You Are Seeking a Safe Place

14.1 My Story — 59
14.3 Bible Verse — 64
14.4 What the Verse Means — 64
14.5 Pray Using Scripture — 64
14.6 Responding to God's Hope — 65
14.7 Takeaway — 65

CHAPTER 15 — 67
Love Me Enough to Let Me Go

15.1 My Story — 67
15.2 We Are the Lord's — 69
15.3 Bible Verse — 70
15.4 What the Verse Means — 70
15.5 Pray Using Scripture — 70
15.6 Responding to God's Hope — 71
15.7 Takeaway — 71

CHAPTER 16
How to Give Your Fears to God — 73

- 16.1 My Story — 73
- 16.2 God's Comfort is Available to You — 74
- 16. 3 Bible Verse — 75
- 16.4 What the Verse Means — 75
- 16.5 Pray Using Scripture — 75
- 16.6 Responding to God's Hope — 76
- 16.7 Takeaway — 76

CHAPTER 17
How to Accept God's Hope — 77

- 17. 1 My Story — 77
- 17.2 Accepting the Hope Available through God — 78
- 17.3 Bible Verse — 78
- 17.4 What the Verse Means — 79
- 17.5 Pray Using Scripture — 79
- 17.6 Responding to God's Hope — 79
- 17.7 Takeaway — 80

CHAPTER 18
Acknowledge God for Real Rest — 81

- 18.1 My Story — 81
- 18.2 Slow Down and Know God — 84
- 18.3 Bible Verse — 84
- 18.4 What the Verse Means — 84
- 18.5 Pray Using Scripture — 84
- 18.6 Responding to God's Hope — 85
- 18.7 Takeaway — 85

CHAPTER 19
I'm Not Going to Sit and Wait to Die — 87

- 19.1 My Story — 87
- 19.2 Not Losing Heart — 89
- 19.3 Bible Verse — 89
- 19.4 What the Verse Means — 89
- 19.5 Pray Using Scripture — 90
- 19.6 Responding to God's Hope — 90
- 19.7 Takeaway — 90

CHAPTER 20 — 91
Faith Frees Me From Fearing Death

- 20.1 My Story — 91
- 20.2 The Value of Giving Thanks — 92
- 20.3 Bible Verse — 93
- 20.4 What the Verse Means — 93
- 20.5 Pray Using Scripture — 93
- 20.6 Responding to God's Hope — 93
- 20.7 Takeaway — 94

CHAPTER 21 — 95
How to Let the Lord Be Your Helper

- 21.1 My Story — 95
- 21.2 The Lord is My Helper — 97
- 21.3 Bible Verse — 97
- 21.4 What the Verse Means — 97
- 21.5 Pray Using Scripture — 97
- 21.6 Responding to God's Hope — 98
- 21.7 Takeaway — 98

CHAPTER 22 — 99
How To Be Comforted During Times of Hardships and Trials

- 22.1 My Story — 99
- 22.2 Developing Compassion for Others — 100
- 22.3 Today's Bible Verses — 101
- 22.4 What the Verses Mean — 101
- 22.5 Pray Using Scripture — 101
- 22.6 Responding to God's Hope — 101
- 22.7 Takeaway — 102

CHAPTER 23 — 103
How to Hang On

- 23.1 My Story — 103
- 23.2 Hang On — 104
- 23.3 Bible Verse — 104
- 23.4 What the Verse Means — 105
- 23.5 Pray Using Scripture — 107
- 23.6 Responding to God's Hope — 107
- 23.7 Takeaway — 107

APPENDIX A *How to Become a Christian*	109
A.1 I Realized I Had a Sin Problem	110
A.2 I Learned There Was a Penalty to be Paid for My Sin	110
A.3 I Learned God Gives Us a Promise	110
A.4 I Learned God Made a Provision for Me	110
A.5 I Prayed to Accept the Gift of Eternal Life Through Jesus	110
A.6 You Can Do Like I Did	111
APPENDIX B *Twenty-one Bible Verses that Teach Us to Wait Upon the Lord*	113
B.1 Wait Upon the Lord	113
B.2 Old Testament Meaning	113
B.3 New Testament Meaning	113
B.4 Twenty-one Bible verses that advise us to wait upon the Lord:	114
APPENDIX C *Twenty Bible Verses to Help with Worry and Anxiety*	117
APPENDIX D *Takeaways*	121
Takeaway from Chapter 1	121
Takeaway from Chapter 2	121
Takeaway from Chapter 3	121
Takeaway from Chapter 4	121
Takeaway from Chapter 5	122
Takeaway from Chapter 6	122
Takeaway from Chapter 7	122
Takeaway from Chapter 8	122
Takeaway from Chapter 9	122
Takeaway from Chapter 10	122
Takeaway from Chapter 11	122
Takeaway from Chapter 12	123
Takeaway from Chapter 13	123
Takeaway from Chapter 14	123
Takeaway from Chapter 15	123
Takeaway from Chapter 16	123
Takeaway from Chapter 17	123
Takeaway from Chapter 18	123

Takeaway from Chapter 19	123
Takeaway from Chapter 20	124
Takeaway from Chapter 21	124
Takeaway from Chapter 22	124
Takeaway from Chapter 23	124

APPENDIX E — 125
Bible Verse Index

APPENDIX F — 135
How to Accept God's Hope

F.1 My Story	135
F.2 I Realized I Had a Sin Problem	136
F.3 I Learned God Gives Us a Promise	136
F.4 I Learned That God Made a Provision for Me	137
F.5 I Prayed to Accept the Gift of Eternal Life Through Jesus	137
F.6 You Can Do Like I Did	137
About the Author	139
HOW TO CONTACT JIMMIE	141

© 2019 Jimmie Aaron Kepler, Ed.D.
All rights reserved

Poetry and Prayer Press

All Bible Verses are from the King James Version (KJV) by Public Domain

This blog is not a substitute for the medical advice of physicians or mental health professionals. The reader should regularly consult a physician in matters relating to his/her or a loved one's health and particularly concerning any symptoms that may require diagnosis or medical attention.

No portion of this material may be reproduced or distributed in any way without the prior written permission of the author, except as allowed by the Copyright Act of the United States of America 1976, as amended.

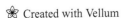 Created with Vellum

INTRODUCTION

When you learn your loved one has a chronic illness, your hopes and dreams may be erased, replaced by feelings of hopelessness. You may feel overwhelmed or even afraid as you look ahead at the day-to-day struggles of caregiving.

Caregiving: Biblical Insights From a Caregiver's Journey offers Biblical guidance and support, helping persons connect with the perfect love which casts out all fear, the love of Jesus Christ.

Each chapter contains Scripture from the Holy Bible, explanation of the verse, application of the Truth to daily living, a prayer using the verse, three directed questions for journaling, and a takeaway.

CHAPTER 1

WHAT'S WITH THE BLOODY SPOT?

1.1 MY STORY

"What's going on? What's with the bloody spot?" I asked, pointing to the half-dollar sized stain on the lower left front of my wife Benita's blouse.

My heart was aching. It looked terrible, scary. I knew this couldn't be good.

Miss Benita gazed down toward the damp crimson. Her eyes looked tired, sad. She said, "It's my mole. It started bleeding."

I recalled the small mole. Forty years earlier, on our wedding night, I had first noticed the growth. Playfully I had kidded her calling it her beauty mark. I found out that was the wrong thing to do. She was sensitive about the mole.

"What's going on?" I asked. I could hear the fear, concern, and the demand for an answer in my voice.

She lifted her eyes, meeting mine. I could see the tears forming. She smiled weakly and then said, "I think I must have scratched or irritated it, maybe at work. It started bleeding a couple of weeks ago. It scabbed over twice, but when I thought it was healing, I would do something to cause the scab to bleed. I thought it would get better. Instead, I think it may get infected. It might become worse, and it's not healing," she said.

Melanoma Cancer, I thought.

"Has Dr. Z looked at it?"

She knows this is bad, I thought.

She shook her head, "No, not yet. I didn't want to mess up our vacation to Colorado and your writer's conference," she answered with a forced smile and then lowered her eyes.

I took her hand, lovingly squeezed it, and hugged her, holding her close. We were out for an afternoon of shopping in a local furniture store and enjoying each other's company.

I nodded and then said, "Let's go home where I can look at it."

She stared at me, our eyes locking for a few seconds. It was as if she was saying I'm sorry, I didn't mean to let it get this bad. She looked sad. Then she nodded.

She knows this is terrible.

We held hands, walked unhurriedly through the store, and to the car. I drove us home. There was a chilling silence in the car.

Once home, I led her to the bedroom and closed the door. She unbuttoned the blouse and removed a blood-soaked gauze bandage. The mole was oozing blood through a cracked, dreadful looking scab.

The mole had grown from the size of an eraser on a number 2 pencil to about the size of a quarter. It had changed from a light brown to a horrible black since I last remembered seeing it.

Melanoma Cancer, I again thought.

"Let's call the dermatologist. I think that's Melanoma Cancer," I said with a seriousness that scared even me.

Miss Benita's lips tightened, and eyes narrowed at hearing the words. She shook slightly and exhaled.

I asked, "Do you want me to call and get you an appointment or do you prefer to call?"

She glanced at herself in the mirror, looking at the mole. "I'll call the dermatologist. Dr. Z will refer me there," she said.

The same day Miss Benita saw the dermatologist an in-office outpatient surgery was performed removing the mole and adjacent tissue. The physician had the test expedited. She called late that night with the biopsy's results.

"I wrote what the doctor told me. She said, 'It's malignant. It is a type of cancer called Melanoma, and it's advanced stage 3. The depth of cancer determines the stage. It's within one centimeter of being stage four.' I know it's bad. I could hear the doctor's quivering voice and her choking back tears. She told me this is serious and could kill me," said a shaken Miss Benita.

The dermatologist gained my wife an appointment with a surgical oncologist. She said I needed to go to the office with my wife. Her finding us an appointment the next morning at 8 AM showed the urgency of the situation. My wife had surgery within a couple of days.

The surgery's findings were terrible. It was Melanoma Cancer. Cancer had spread to the lymph nodes.

The oncological surgeon removed thirty-four lymph nodes. The physician told me the five-year survival rate for these findings was less than ten percent.

While my wife was still in recovery at the hospital, the surgeon told us some treatment options and that when not if cancer recurred, they would reclassify it to Melanoma Cancer stage 4 and would be terminal.

There was no cure. She said death was the ultimate destination of this journey, barring God's intervention or a new pharmaceutical breakthrough.

I knew Melanoma Cancer stage 3 was too big for me to handle. I didn't realize it, but I had already moved into a new role as a caregiver. The future my wife and I had planned together had suddenly changed. We would have no retirement years to share. Death would call on Miss Benita before then.

Our hopes and dreams vanished. Despair and hopelessness replaced them. I was overwhelmed just thinking about the day-to-day struggles of caregiving. I faced the fear of the unknown.

So many questions flooded my mind. Would my wife survive? How long would she live? What would be the quality of her life and mine? Could we pay the medical bills? How much help was she going to need from me daily? Could I be strong and help her? How was this going to affect our day jobs?

I also had concerns for our three grown children and granddaughter. What I needed was hope.

This book shares the hope Christians have and the hope that my wife and I exercised through our faith in Jesus Christ. It shares my journey as a caregiver.

"Caregiving: Biblical Insights from a Caregiver's Journey" offers Biblical guidance and support, helping you in your role as caregiver. It will help you connect with the perfect love which casts out all fear, the love of Jesus Christ.

The day I noticed the bloody spot on Miss Benita's blouse, my wife and I prayed together. We shared I love you and claimed, Psalm 56:3 (KJV), "What time I am afraid I will trust in thee" and 1 Peter 5:7 "Cast all your cares on the Lord for He careth for you."

This story does not have an Earthly happily ever after ending. My wife lived 1001 days from her first surgery. Then she died.

The faith we both had in Jesus Christ allowed us to face each day with hope.

Yes, even with our hope we had because of our Christian faith, we still were afraid. However, our trust in Jesus Christ carried us through the process, moving us from fear to a calmness that could only come from God. That my wife was a Christian gave us a real-world spiritual happily ever after ending. She is in heaven today, and one day, since I am also a Christian, I will join her there.

1.2 IT'S OKAY TO BE AFRAID

Part of caring for a person with a chronic illness understands that fear of the unknown and fear of the journey you are beginning is normal. It's a scary assignment. When you're a caregiver, it's okay to be afraid.

You also need to learn to accept the hope for the caregiver that's available through Jesus Christ. The hope available through the love of Jesus Christ will help you face and handle the fears you will encounter in your journey of caregiving.

1.3 BIBLE VERSE

1 John 4:18 King James Version of the Holy Bible (KJV), "There is no fear in love; but perfect love casteth out fear: because fear hath torment. He that feareth is not made perfect in love."

1.4 WHAT THE VERSE MEANS

John says that perfect love produces courage in the day of judgment. It casts out fear.

How does the perfect love of Jesus Christ accomplish the casting out of fear? Perfect love casts out fear because it produces a likeness to Christ.

There is another way in which love produces boldness. It does this by casting out fear. The entrance of perfect love through Jesus Christ is for fear a "cease and desist" letter. It is an order to quit.

When love arrives, it brings hand in hand with itself courage.

Boldness is the companion of love, only when love is perfect. Only professing Christians can experience this perfect love of God, a love that casts out fear.

As Believer's in Jesus Christ, we can face the future, including being the caregiver of a loved one with a chronic illness, and even confront their death with the peace that only comes from Christ's perfect love.

If you are not a Christian, accepting Jesus Christ as your Savior is a prerequisite to getting God's peace.

Appendix A explains how to become a Christian. You can trust Jesus Christ today.

See Appendix A at the back of this book for information on How to Become a Christian.

1.5 PRAY USING SCRIPTURE

- Lord Jesus, thank You that there is no fear in love; but perfect love casts out fear.
- Heavenly Father, help me keep my mind focused on You and Your love for me.
- God, help me remove any concerns I may have as I look to the future by turning them over to You.
- Provide Your grace to meet the challenges I encounter daily. I cannot travel this journey alone but can with You.
- Help me know with no doubt that as a Believer in Jesus Christ, my ultimate future is in Heaven.
- Help my loved one to trust in Jesus Christ as their Lord and Savior if they are not a Christian.

- If my loved one is not a Christian, prepare their heart to hear the Gospel and to accept Christ as Savior.

1.6 RESPONDING TO GOD'S HOPE

1. List two examples of times you have been afraid (Psalm 56:3 and 1 Peter 5:7).
2. Remember two times you have trusted in God since the diagnosis of your loved one's chronic illness (Psalm 56:3 and 1 Peter 5:7).
3. List two cares or concerns you are facing. Cast (or give) those cares to the Lord, remembering that "He careth for you." (1 Peter 5:7).

1.7 TAKEAWAY

Part of caring for a person with a chronic illness understands that fear of the unknown and fear of the journey is normal.

CHAPTER 2

HOW TO BE COURAGEOUS

2.1 MY STORY

One of the first thoughts I had when my wife received the diagnosis that she had stage three Melanoma Cancer was how am I going to care for her and love her unconditionally until she dies.

I knew the Melanoma Cancer was going to kill her unless God intervened. I wondered if she would follow the doctor's orders. Would my wife let me help her? How would she react? Could I handle being her caregiver?

In time, they answered all the questions. The solutions didn't happen in one day. There was some give and take.

My spouse had to have a heart to heart with me along the way, which included telling me to back off and give her some space as I was smothering her with kindness and care.

She didn't need me reacting as if every minor event she encountered was a life or death situation. I learned what she needed was for me to be there. She desired my steady presence.

A simple example was when I had a ball game on the television, and she came into the room I would change channels on the TV to her favorite HGTV program. I stayed in the room with her instead of going to the bedroom and continuing the ballgame. If I were cleaning, doing other housework, or even reading, I would stop, give her my attention and be with her.

In her last days of hospice care, she told me how much my just being there meant to her. She said I could get the house spotless after she was in heaven, but until then she needed the ministry of my presence. She needed me to be courageous as I spent time with her.

2.2 HOW TO BE COURAGEOUS

Part of caring for a person with a chronic illness understands how to be courageous in the Lord.

Caring for a person with a chronic illness is a scary daily challenge for both the person with the disease, their family, and you as the caregiver. Through Jesus Christ, we can be courageous.

How can we do this?

We cannot do this in our strength. Daily the Lord Jesus, our God goes with the Christian. We need to remember He goes with us. We need the Lord to strengthen us.

Today's Scripture tells us the Lord will not leave or forsake the Believer in Jesus Christ.

2.3 BIBLE VERSE

Deuteronomy 31:6 (KJV), "Be strong and of a good courage, fear not, nor be afraid of them: for the Lord thy God, he it is that doth go with thee; he will not fail thee, nor forsake thee."

2.4 WHAT THE VERSE MEANS

Because Christians have God with them, they should be of good courage. The courage comes from their confident assurance in God, which faith gives. This faith in Christ allows us to face each day bravely, knowing through Him we shall have the ultimate victory.

2.5 PRAY USING SCRIPTURE

- Heavenly Father, please help me and my family to continue to be courageous in the face of this illness.
- Holy Spirit, I ask for Your comfort. Help me to not fear or be in dread of the challenges I face as a caregiver. Help me not to grow weary.
- Thank You for letting me know it is the Lord our God who goes with me and that He will not leave me or forsake me.
- I pray my family and loved ones' would confess faith in Jesus Christ, where they too can experience the comfort available to Christians.

2.6 RESPONDING TO GOD'S HOPE

1. What are two areas that you are fearful of failing in as you care for your loved one? Name them.
2. Take the two items you identified in question one. Admit your fears to God. Ask God for the faith you need to face fear courageously.
3. Realize that God has entrusted you already with your loved one's care. He's put them under your supervision; God will equip you for the daily challenges you face. Thank God for the confidence He has placed in you, and for the way, He helps you daily as you care for your loved one.

2.7 TAKEAWAY

Part of learning to care for a person with a chronic illness understands how to rely on the Lord.

CHAPTER 3

YOU HAVE PERMISSION TO CRY

3.1 MY STORY

"I removed the tumor. The tests showed it has spread to your wife's lymph nodes. I removed thirty-four lymph nodes," said the surgical oncologist.

I stared at the doctor. She was slowly becoming out of focus as I became teary-eyed. I knew the initial diagnosis of Stage 3 Melanoma Cancer was terrible. Melanoma Cancer spreading into the lymph nodes was terrible. I knew this would kill my wife. Even though I was trying hard not to, I started sobbing.

The surgeon then said the words I needed to hear. She said, "It's okay to cry."

She took me in her arms, and I wept.

With her four simple words, I stopped pretending to be a macho man, let down my guard, and let the emotions of the moment take over. She had given me permission to cry.

Today wouldn't be the last time sobbing would overcome me. I would cry many more times over the next thirty-four months. Even now, over one year since my wife's passing, the crying returns from time to time.

Remember, you have permission to cry.

The Bible tells of Jesus crying when Lazarus died. The Heavenly Father cares about our tears. Today's Bible verse tells what God's word says about crying.

3.2 TEARS ARE NORMAL

Part of caring for a person with a chronic illness realizes that tears are normal. Caring for a loved one will bring tears. It's okay to cry. Even Jesus wept (John 11:35 KJV, "Jesus wept.").

3.3 BIBLE VERSE

Psalm 56:8-9 (KJV), "Thou tellest my wanderings: put thou my tears into thy bottle: are they not in thy book? When I cry unto thee, then shall mine enemies turn back: this I know; for God is for me."

3.4 WHAT THE VERSES MEAN

Why would God keep tears in a bottle?

The idea behind the keeping of "tears in a bottle" is a remembrance. King David, the writer of these verses, is expressing a deep trust in God. He knows God remembers his sorrow. He knows God remembers his tears.

King David also is sure the God will never forget about him. David is confident that God is on his side.

3.5 PRAY USING SCRIPTURE

- Heavenly Father, thank You for making us where we can cry and experience the emotional release of the resulting tears. Teach me to understand and accept that my tears help me identify and help me deal with my feelings.
- Lord Jesus, thank You for letting me know crying is okay.
- Almighty God, it is comforting to know that You notice and keep track of my tears.
- I turn the sorrow concerning the chronic illness of my loved one and my ability to care for them over to You. You are Yahweh-Rapha (God, that heals).
- I pray that my family and I would feel the freedom to cry out to You God and let the tears flow when we need the release.
- Let my family and friends would be supportive, loving, and understanding during the times the tears flow.
- I pray I would hold on to God during these times without questioning. Help me accept God's comfort.
- Help me have the confidence of King David, the author of these verses, and say with him - for God is for me.

3.6 RESPONDING TO GOD'S HOPE

1. Have you given yourself and your loved one's permission to cry? Remember, it's okay to shed tears. Share with your family members that sometimes you cry. Sharing your weeping will permit them to do the same. Sometimes they need to cry. List some times you have cried.
2. Remember that God will not forget about your loved one. He does not forget about you or the other caregivers. Thank God for remembering you and not deserting you. List two examples of when God remembered you.
3. What is the first concern you think of for caring for your loved

one? Tell God what that concern is and remember, it's okay to cry. Tears are normal.

3.7 TAKEAWAY

God gives you permission to cry. Your Heavenly Father even collects your tears in a bottle.

CHAPTER 4

HOW TO REST IN GOD

4.1 MY STORY

You may be like my late wife when she was battling Stage Four Melanoma Cancer. She found herself exhausted. She needed rest.

My daily caregiving of my wife also left me weary. Like my wife, I needed rest.

The managing of my wife's schedule required a skill set that even an air traffic controller would envy. First, she had the never ending visits to her primary medical team. The army of medical doctors included the primary care physician, surgical oncologist, managing oncologist, dermatologist, gastroenterologist, thyroid doctor, cardiologist (the heart must be healthy enough for the treatments) and radiologist. These physicians did the routine checks, prescribed the medications, treatments, performed biopsies, surgery and ordered the tests.

A group of medical technicians did the grunt work of tests and treatment procedures. In this category was blood work, PET scans, CAT scans, MRIs, days and weeks of radiation treatments and the lymphedema therapy.

At home, my wife did months of daily chemotherapy prescription medications, spent hours waiting for UPS or FedEx to deliver the refrigerated prescriptions from the exotic, super expensive pharmacy, did 24/7/365 lymphedema therapy at home with the machine that sounded like Darth Vader with a sleeve that looked like the nose of Snuffleupagus on Sesame Street.

Added to these challenges was managing her work schedule to maintain health insurance. These alone were enough to have her constantly exhausted. Unfortunately, more daily challenges were adding to her fatigue.

My wife's eating schedule controlled her life. She had to take the prescription medications and then wait two hours to eat or eat and wait several hours before she could take the medications. The routine dictated the time of day when she woke and went to bed.

You get the picture and can relate. Like my wife, you get tired. Yes, the patient gets tired. The caregiver also gets worn down. The caregiver makes sure the loved one stays on schedule and task.

As the caregiver, you need to rest. You need God.

4.2 RESTING IN THE LORD

Part of caring for a person with a chronic illness understands the need for resting in the Lord.

Caregiving for a loved one with a chronic illness can leave you tired and weary. I am talking about becoming bone tired. I am talking about the type of fatigue that vacations or even a sabbatical cannot cure.

4.3 BIBLE VERSE

Exodus 33:14 (KJV), "My presence will go with you, and I will give you rest."

4.4 WHAT THE VERSE MEANS

The Lord is telling Moses that God will go with him. The Lord will give him rest. He is informing Moses that everything will ultimately be fine for him.

For the caregiver, this doesn't mean that your loved one will be healed in this life. Finally, healing may not happen until heaven.

The application for the Believer in Christ is the Lord also goes with us, gives us rest, and promises to sustain us during our caregiving journey.

4.5 PRAY USING SCRIPTURE

- Heavenly Father, thank you for Your presence going with us.
- Lord Jesus, thank you for the rest You give us.
- God, we ask to experience Your rest again this day.
- Let us use Sundays as the day of rest and worship.

4.6 RESPONDING TO GOD'S HOPE

1. Remember, a recent time you felt God's presence. What were you doing? Recall how you felt His presence.
2. Ask God to go with you and be with you today as you work and go about your caregiving responsibilities.
3. Are you getting enough rest? Do you read your Bible regularly? Are you getting enough sleep? Are you taking time to be still and listen to God?

4.7 TAKEAWAY

God goes with us both sustaining and provides the rest we need.

CHAPTER 5

HOW TO HAVE REAL DELIVERANCE

5.1 MY STORY

Miss Benita's left arm had swollen up. The wrist and hand also puffed up. Both were getting noticeably larger day by day.

My wife called the surgical oncologist for instructions on managing the swelling. This surgeon referred my wife to the managing oncologist.

One day shortly after the phone calls, my wife greeted me with additional information. She said, "I have lymphedema."

"They removed thirty-four of your lymph nodes last June when you had your Melanoma Cancer surgery. The lymph node removal and lymphoma seem related. Am I right?" I queried.

"Don't look so smug. You don't know everything," Miss Benita replied playfully.

"It looks and sounds serious," I said, staring at her left arm and hand.

"It is."

She explained to me that lymphedema is a condition of localized fluid retention and tissue swelling caused by a compromised lymphatic system. In her case, the cause was complications from her cancer surgery.

"Can they treat it? What are they going to do?"

"I have an appointment with a lymphedema therapist later this week."

She saw the lymphedema therapist who performed two weeks of massage by hand of her arm, wrist, and hand. They followed the message therapy with a lymphedema therapy machine being delivered to our home for home treatment.

For the next twenty-eight months she would attach herself to the device for an hour a day to reduce the swelling in the arm.

And no, she didn't have to do the therapy the rest of her life. Five months before her death, the brain tumor she developed had an unexpected positive side effect. A combination of massive amounts of steroids taken to reduce swelling in the brain also reduced swelling in the arm. It overjoyed Miss Benita not having to do the lymphedema therapy.

The lymphedema was just the first of six addition afflictions my sweet wife experienced following her initial surgery.

Somehow, she maintained a Godly, optimistic attitude through it all. I can testify the Lord Jesus delivered her out of it all.

As her caregiver, I helped her stay on schedule, encouraged her, and picked up some of her former household responsibilities where she could go to the treatments without feeling guilty.

5.2 DELIVERANCE FOR THE BELIEVER IS IN JESUS CHRIST

Part caring for a person with a chronic illness understands God's deliverance for the Believer in Jesus Christ. The Bible does not flatter us with the false hope that goodness will secure us from trouble. Instead, the Bible warns us over and over to expect tribulation while we are in this body.

Our afflictions come unannounced from all directions. The challenges are many, but with Jesus Christ, we can face each day.

There is no promise the challenges, problems, illness, or disease will go away in this lifetime. However, the Lord will guide us through or lift us out of them.

5.3 BIBLE VERSE

Psalm 34:19, "Many are the afflictions of the righteous, but the Lord delivers him out of them all."

5.4 WHAT THE VERSE MEANS

We either have faced, are confronting, or will experience afflictions and trials. Suffering is an unchangeable fact.

There is good news. God's mercies are more numerous than the afflictions and trials. His wisdom more wondrous than the sufferings and trials. God's power is more miraculous than the hardships and trials. God will give us the grace we need to face them, and God will deliver us.

5.5 PRAY USING SCRIPTURE

- Heavenly Father, I know the afflictions of the righteous are many.
- Lord Jesus, I find some comfort in knowing hardships and trials are the norms.
- I confess I don't like the difficulties and trials, but trust in You.
- God our Father, I thank You for the promise of deliverance.

5.6 RESPONDING TO GOD'S HOPE

1. What new challenges is your loved one facing?
2. How can you help them as they navigate the new challenges?
3. Have you asked God for the grace you need for the problems? Give God the glory for meeting your needs when he provides the needed grace. Acknowledge his presence and activity in your loved one and your lives.

5.7 TAKEAWAY

During our life we face many challenges. With Jesus, we can face each day.

CHAPTER 6

ANY DELAY COULD BE LIFE THREATENING

6.1 MY STORY

"I need your decision on starting radiation treatment. What have you decided?" asked the surgical oncologist.

"Not today. I can't decide today," said my wife with angst in her voice.

It was apparent they overwhelmed her with everything.

"Any delay could be life-threatening at the worst and potentially life-shortening. You need to decide on when you want to start treatments," pressed the oncologist.

My wife rolled her tired eyes. She was less than a month from the initial Melanoma Cancer surgery and the removal of both the cancerous area and thirty-four lymph nodes. She had a swollen left arm, wrist, and hand. Lymphedema therapy had just started that week.

Miss Benita glanced at me for help.

"Can you go over the treatment options for us one more time? We'll then go home and have some time to meditate and pray about what she'll do next. We understand the urgency for beginning treatment," I said.

My wife exhaled slowly, smiled, and nodded.

This time it was the young surgical oncologist who rolled her eyes. She nodded and dutifully repeated the options. She concluded with a "Let me know soon what you are or are not going to do. While selecting no treatment is an option, not having the radiation increases the chances of recurrence. If it recurs," she added with a strong emphasis, "the Melanoma Cancer will be terminal. There will be no treatment or cure. You will die."

"Thank you. We'll let you know in a few days," I said as I saw Miss Benita flinch. On the inside, I was mad at how the doctor had restated the obvious — "If it recurs, it will be terminal. There will be no treatment or cure. You will die."

On the hour drive home, my wife slept. She was tired and weary. Over the next few days together, we prayed, read Scripture, and then she said, "Call the doctor and find out who I need to contact to schedule the radiation."

I called the surgical oncologist, getting the contact information. Benita called and set up an appointment.

God's timing amazed me. The radiation doctor had a patient cancel an appointment. If she could come now, they could get her in that very afternoon. If we had rushed and said yes to treatment four days earlier, radiation treatments would not have started for nearly two weeks. Praying and seeking God's guidance allowed treatment to begin almost immediately.

I firmly believe seeking God in her decisions is one reason she lived over two-years longer than the initial projections.

It's another example of my wife's Godly wisdom and God's faithfulness.

6.2 HEARING GOD'S VOICE

Part of caring for a person with a chronic or terminal illness is listening until we hear God's voice.

When we face a chronic disease too often, we rush in and try to accomplish everything in our power. Manage this. Plan that. We listen to this aunt or that special trusted friend. We may hear conflicting recommendations from our healing team, that is the doctors, ministers, social workers, counselors, and other caregivers.

While wise counsel is right, we also need to seek God and listen to his voice. We do this through prayer, Bible reading, and listening to sermons.

We need to encourage our loved one to do the same.

Sometimes we are in such a rush to get to a solution or get things under control that we miss hearing from "The Great Physician." We need to remember the words of Psalm 46:10 (KJV), "Be still, and know that I am God:"

Sometimes we need to sit and be still before we can hear God.

6.3 BIBLE VERSE

Psalm 143:8 (KJV) "Cause me to hear thy lovingkindness in the morning; for in thee do I trust: cause me to know the way wherein I should walk; for I lift up my soul unto thee."

6.4 WHAT THE VERSE MEANS

As we face trials and hardships, we can find ourselves overwhelmed. When we become inundated by fear, grief, depression, and self-pity, it becomes hard to hear God.

Psalm 143:8 reminds us to spend time with God, to begin our day with God. As Christians, we can trust God. Ask Him to guide us. Stop, slow down, and take time for God. We need to read the Bible and meditate on His Word. We need to listen, to hear sermons, hymns, and listen to God's still small voice answering our prayers.

6.5 PRAY USING SCRIPTURE

- Heavenly Father, draw me to You in the morning where I can hear Your righteousness.
- Lord Jesus, I place my trust in You. Help me to always put all my faith in You.
- I ask Your Holy Spirit to speak to my spirit and to guide me in the way I should walk.
- Lift my soul unto You.
- I pray for myself, my spouse, our children, and grandchildren to be drawn to You, to experience You and choose to attend worship services where we can hear Your word preached.

6.6 RESPONDING TO GOD'S HOPE

1. Are you including God in your decision-making process? James 1:5 (KJV) reminds us, "If any of you lack wisdom, let him ask of God, that giveth to all men liberally, and upbraideth not; and it shall be given him."
2. Are you listening for Gods still small voice?
3. Are you slowing down and waiting on God?

6.7 TAKEAWAY

We need to spend time with God. We do this by reading the Bible, listening to Hymns and spiritual songs, listening to sermons, and by prayer and meditation. Spending time with God helps us make Godly decisions and helps us to wait upon the Lord and His timing.

CHAPTER 7

THE THERAPEUTIC VALUE OF ROMANTIC COMEDIES

7.1 MY STORY

There is nothing funny about a spouse having a chronic or terminal illness. There indeed isn't anything comical about caring for them and all the nuisances involved with the daily routine.

Over the years I had heard time and time again that opposites attract. My experience would agree with the statement. Many times I have been told I am the least spontaneous person alive.

Maybe my living my life structured like a German railroad schedule or the fact I grew up in a career military family and then was a US Army officer helped influence me in this arena. My wife enjoyed the structure of routine but also loved the unexpected blessings of life. Where I needed a to-do list and schedule for my day and struggled when I had my day disrupted with change, she embraced the unexpected.

I also am a very stoic person. Again, being a military officer affected me in this area. I believe nearly twenty-years of full-time Christian ministry also had me being the rock of stability in difficult situations. I was the steady influence, the calm in the storm for so many. It allowed me to officiate funerals of friends and even my parents with a solemn seriousness that my wife sometimes hated and caused others to refer to me as a robot-man.

I remember the surgical oncologist strongly encouraging me to lighten up. She said my serious all the time attitude was contagious. My constant seriousness was gloomy and the incorrect disposition for my wife to catch.

The doctor added attitude is crucial when dealing with a chronic illness like my wife's cancer. The cheerfulness of mind does good, like a medicine for the body. Our outlook contributes to the restoration or preservation of bodily health and vigor.

Medical science tells us the red blood cells, most white blood cells, and platelets are produced in the bone marrow, the soft fatty tissue inside bone cavities. Proverbs 17:22 (KJV) teaches, "A poor spirit/attitude 'drieth the bones' which produces the needed cells."

The surgical oncologist encouraged me to watch romantic comedies, funny situation comedies, and even some comedy specials with my wife. She said they would get us both laughing. It would help me lighten my mood. It would help with my wife's healing. She said there is therapeutic value in watching romantic comedies.

The medical doctor questioned my expectation of the value of the prescribed treatments, asking if I was already given over to my wife's death to cancer. She said it was too early to give up hope. She said those with a more positive attitude live longer. Her little talk helped me to recalibrate my thinking and adjust my outlook. She said I should embrace the time I would have with my spouse. Maybe my making that slight change in viewpoint contributed to my spouse's living almost two years longer than first expected. Only God knows if it did.

By the way, we can learn a lot if we read our Bible.

CAREGIVING

7.2 LEARNING TO LAUGH

Part of caring for a person with a chronic illness is learning to laugh.

7.3 BIBLE VERSE

Proverbs 17:22 (KJV), "A merry heart doeth good like a medicine: but a broken spirit drieth the bones."

7.4 WHAT THE VERSE MEANS

Our attitude is crucial when dealing with a chronic illness. The cheerfulness of our mind does good, like a medicine for the body. Our opinion contributes to the restoration or preservation of bodily health and vigor.

7.5 PRAY USING SCRIPTURE

- Lord Jesus, help me enjoy the funny things that happen in life.
- Heavenly Father, help me take life one day at a time.
- God, help me, and my family and friends to not dwell on the seriousness of the chronic illness, but help us live life to the fullest as we know You hold the future.

7.6 RESPONDING TO GOD'S HOPE

1. How is your attitude? Do you need an attitude change? If so, God can help. Ask Him.
2. Are you remaining affirming and confident? Remember, your outlook and attitude are catching. I'm not talking about some false it's going to be all better attitude but a realistic today is going to be a good day attitude — and I'm going to do my best to make it a good day approach instead of a gloom and doom outlook.

3. What can you do to bring joy and laughter today? Is there a favorite movie or comedy series you could watch together?

7.7 TAKEAWAY

Having a positive attitude helps as you care for your loved one. It helps both you and your loved one.

CHAPTER 8

HOW TO USE YOUR REMAINING TIME

8.1 MY STORY

"How long..."

I asked the question doctors dread to hear. How long will my wife live?

I had spoken those words to the physician when my mother had her kidney transplant. Those two words I repeated when I took my ninety-year-old father to the emergency room and found out he had suffered a major heart attack that would take his life in hours. I echoed the words when my wife had Melanoma Cancer surgery and had thirty-four lymph nodes removed because the disease had spread into them.

With my spouse, I remember the oncologist giving the five-year survival rate odds, which were very depressing. She emphasized enjoying the now. The doctor strongly stressed if cancer recurred it would be terminal. She said, "Live for today. Enjoy every day."

Less than six months later, the Melanoma Cancer returned. My wife lived another two years and two months after the recurrence. She survived nearly two years longer than what we were told to expect.

I worked hard to make each day she lived a positive experience. I also took her on a multi-week "bucket list" trip where we had quality time together.

The trip was challenging as I had to get a refrigerator for our car for her prescription chemotherapy medications. Daily, I also had to pack and unpack a cumbersome lymphedema therapy machine. My wife had to sit for an hour every day hooked to the device to control swelling in her left arm, wrist, and hand.

My point is we well used the time available. I made sure she saw her sisters multiple times. I made sure our grown children were engaged in her life.

God was gracious and gave her 1001 days from the first surgery. He also gave me the patience and desire to serve her.

The hope we both had through Jesus Christ allowed us to face each day with hope.

8.2 USE THE TIME GOD HAS GIVEN YOU

Part of caring for a person with a chronic illness is learning to use the time God has given you. The Bible teaches God has the days of our lives numbered. Here are five examples:

1. Job 14:5 King James Version (KJV), "Seeing his days are determined, the number of his months are with thee, thou hast appointed his bounds that he cannot pass;"
2. Job 21:21 (KJV), "For what does he care for his household after him, When the number of his months is cut off?"
3. Psalm 31:15 (KJV), "My times are in Your hand; Deliver me from the hand of my enemies and from those who persecute me."
4. Psalm 139:16 (KJV), "Your eyes have seen my unformed substance; And in Your book were all written The days that

were ordained for me, When as yet there was not one of them."
5. Ecclesiastes 3:2 (KJV), "A time to give birth and a time to die; A time to plant and a time to uproot what is planted."

8.3 BIBLE VERSE

Psalm 39:4 (KJV), "Lord, make me to know mine end, and the measure of my days, what it is: that I may know how frail I am."

8.4 WHAT THE VERSE MEANS

The verse shares thoughts concerning the psalmist meditations on human life. He reflects on life's brevity, life's vanity, and life's sorrows.

He wonders why life was so short. Why was it so vain? Why was it so full of pain?

8.5 PRAY USING SCRIPTURE

- Father in heaven, thank You for reminding me of how brief my time on earth will be. Help me use the days I have with my loved one to the fullest.
- Lord Jesus, thank You for reminding me You are in control of the length of a person's life. Help me trust You know what is best for me.
- God, help me remember how fleeting my life is and to live my days to Your honor and Your glory.

8.6 RESPONDING TO GOD'S HOPE

1. Are you helping your loved live the remaining days of their

life to the fullest? What can you do today to make today a good day for your loved one?
2. What can you do to encourage friends and family to engage with your chronically or terminally ill loved one?
3. Make sure you include rest in the management of your one's time. What can you do today to make sure you take time to rest?

8.7 TAKEAWAY

The Bible teaches God has numbered our days. We need to live each day to the fullest.

CHAPTER 9

THE SOURCE OF REAL PEACE

9.1 MY STORY

I thought I was Superman. Belief that I could handle anything that would come my way in caring for my wife as she battled Melanoma Cancer filled me.

I was wrong.

Over Mother's Day Weekend in May 2016, my wife started an eleven-month treatment with prescription chemotherapy medications. In less than twenty-four hours of taking her first dosage, her temperature was 104-degrees. She was disoriented, non-communicative, and near death. I was scared and felt helpless.

All three of my grown children were home for the Mother's Day Weekend. My wife's two sisters had flown in from out of state to visit. They had good reason to come.

My wife's PET Scan in late April had shown Melanoma Cancer had spread. It was in her left shoulder, lungs, between her lungs, in her thyroid, neck, pelvic area, right thigh, and in almost every area of the body except the brain. The oncologist said my wife would have weeks to months to live without the new chemotherapy prescription medications.

Miss Benita reluctantly agreed to the chemotherapy meds. Within hours of taking them, she wished she hadn't. She was sure death would be better than dealing with the sickness she was now experiencing.

I remembered the managing oncologist's instructions as she started the medications. He had said she might experience elevated temperature. Her temperature was 104-degrees plus. Her fever was extreme. He also said nausea was common. Her nausea was endless vomiting. I was told to call the doctor first before taking her to an emergency room at the hospital or calling 911 if she experienced these side-effects.

I called the doctor. He gave detailed instructions. I felt like I was now a critical care registered nurse. I felt overwhelmed, incompetent, scared, and responsible for my wife. He had me make sure she stayed hydrated. We stopped the chemo meds for a few days. We adjusted the dosages and their administration.

During this time my wife's oldest sister's faith in God, calm demeanor and trust in my caring for her sister guided me through the valley of the shadow of death I knew my wife was walking through. Somehow my bride's body adjusted to the meds. They were miracle drugs. Her adjusting to them was equally miraculous.

Within six-weeks, the PET Scan showed no traces of the Melanoma Cancer. The next seventeen months, all scans and tests showed no Melanoma Cancer. The cancer stayed in remission from then until December 7, 2017, when the diagnosis of a brain tumor changed everything. My wife never had Melanoma Cancer recur anywhere in her body except in the brain. Unfortunately, the prescription chemo meds could not cross the blood-brain barrier into the brain. This is a natural barrier designed by God to protect the brain.

During the process with the chemotherapy prescription medications, I saw an amazing peace descend on both my wife and me. Yes, it was a God thing. But it also was a family thing. Having sister's in law that prayed and believed was a blessing. My children's belief in my ability to care for their mother also helped. I confess I wasn't short of hubris in this area.

God's giving me peace of mind and an ability to keep on keeping on was the key. God is faithful. I can testify that I cried out to God, and He was there to walk with me through caring for my wife.

9.2 REAL PEACE COMES FROM GOD

Part of caring for a person with a chronic illness understands that real peace comes from God. Living to care for a person with a chronic disease can leave us overwhelmed.

The endless stream of questions from well-meaning family, friends, acquaintances, and coworkers drains us. We find ourselves emotionally and physically exhausted. We need more than rest. What we need is peace.

As we learn to care for a person with a chronic illness, we realize that real peace comes from God.

9.3 BIBLE VERSE

John 14:27 (KJV), "Peace I leave with you, my peace I give unto you: not as the world giveth, give I unto you. Let not your heart be troubled, neither let it be afraid."

9.4 WHAT THE VERSE MEANS

The verse uses the Jewish form of greeting and blessing. Indeed, the hearers understand this wish for peace. Jesus wishes them the same serenity of soul as he experiences. He leaves the availability of this peace with them.

Jesus lets them know his words are not idle or meaningless. He means what he says. His words are true.

Because his words are factual, we should not fear the future. No matter how difficult the challenges are that you face, stand firm. Remember Jesus paid the price for your comfort, salvation, and redemption.

9.5 PRAYER USING SCRIPTURE

- Heavenly Father, thank You for the gift of peace.
- Lord, I pray my heart would not be troubled.
- I pray I would not fear as I continue the battle against the chronic illness.

9.6 RESPONDING TO GOD'S HOPE

1. Have you asked God for peace of mind? Why not ask now?
2. Have you turned your fears over to the Lord? He's listening even now. I encourage you to list them. God will hear you.
3. Being afraid is normal. Thank God for giving you the ability to feel and care.

9.7 TAKEAWAY

Real peace comes from God.

CHAPTER 10

HOW TO HAVE REAL DIRECTION FOR YOUR LIFE

10.1 MY STORY

I was always amazed at the child-like faith my wife showed in the Lord Jesus Christ. Her faith reminded me of a bumper sticker frequently seen in the late 1960s and early 1970s. It just stated, "God said it, I believe it, and that settles it."

As she confronted cancer, she regularly would quote Job 14:5-7 King James Version (KJV), "Seeing his days are determined, the number of his months are with thee, thou hast appointed his bounds that he cannot pass; Turn from him, that he may rest, till he shall accomplish, as a hireling, his day."

She would comment that she was getting the recommended treatment the medical team suggested. She knew the team of physicians were part of the healing team and God's plan.

Then she would add, "You know, God has my days numbered. He knew from the beginning of time when I was going to be born. He also knows when He is calling me home."

She saw no need to worry about doing this or trying that to squeeze an extra day of life. She knew her Heavenly Father already had it all worked out. Acceptance of God's plan for her life occurred without question.

I pray my faith in God could show an equal trust in God.

10.2 THY WORD

Part of caring for a person with a chronic illness understands the power of God's Word.

This chapter's verse, Jeremiah 15:16, is a reminder of the power and guidance of God's word, the Holy Bible. Psalm 119:105 (KJV) helps explain part of the purpose of God's word. It reads, "Thy word is a lamp unto my feet, and a light unto my path."

10.3 BIBLE VERSE

Jeremiah 15:16 (KJV), "Thy words were found, and I did eat them; and thy word was unto me the joy and rejoicing of mine heart: for I am called by thy name, O Lord God of hosts."

10.4 WHAT THE VERSE MEANS

The verse reflects Jeremiah's call to the office of prophet. He had not sought or expected to be a prophet. Likewise, God calls us to follow him as Believers of Jesus Christ.

As Jeremiah mentions eating the words of God, he is expressing the close relationship between him and God that comes from reading, hearing, and consuming the word of God.

Jeremiah concludes the passage, telling us he is called by God's name. It is a reminder that God set him apart and ordained him to be a prophet.

CAREGIVING

Likewise, as a Believer in Jesus Christ, God has selected you and you, as Jeremiah, are required to respond to God having selected you.

10.5 PRAY USING SCRIPTURE

- Heavenly Father, thank You for the Bible, Your word.
- Lord God, help me listen to, meditate, and memorize Your Word, and allow Your Word to sustain me.
- Your Word brings joy to my heart.
- Lord Jesus, that You for selecting me.

10.6 RESPONDING TO GOD'S HOPE

1. Are you trusting God for your tomorrows?
2. Are you reading and applying the Bible to your everyday living?
3. Have you considered offering to read the Bible to your loved one? You can just ask, "Is okay for me to share a short Bible passage that really spoke to me?"

10.7 TAKEAWAY

God's Word is perfect. His Word provides direction for your life.

CHAPTER 11

HOW TO TRUST GOD

11.1 MY STORY

In August 2016, my wife Benita and I took a lengthy "bucket list" trip. In our forty-plus years of marriage, she had never been to the northeastern USA. She had heard stories from my early teens when I lived in New England as a military brat. She also had never been to New York or the middle Atlantic states.

The trip wasn't easy. Even with my wife's terminal Melanoma Cancer her employer initially said no to her being off work for multiple weeks of vacation even though she had sufficient accrued vacation days. My day job also lacked compassion. We both found the situation frustrating as we had more days of leave accumulated than needed for the trip. Finally, both employers agreed to let us off work.

The trip required a small refrigerator for the car as her chemotherapy prescription medications needed refrigeration. The large lymphedema therapy machine had to be unloaded and loaded each day along with scheduling time for her to do an hour's therapy per day.

Many days it would be as later than 10 AM before we could get checked out of our hotel. Most days 5 PM found us checked into the hotel for the evening. When you drive those few hours in a day, it takes a long time to travel the over 2,200 miles from Dallas, Texas to Northern Maine.

Our lengthy trip included stops at cool places like Niagara Falls, and Ben and Jerry's Ice Cream Factory just outside of Burlington, Vermont. We visited university campuses like Dartmouth, Harvard, MIT, Bowdoin College, Brown, Yale, Virginia Military Institute, Washington and Lee Universities, and their libraries. She saw where I attended junior high school in Portsmouth, New Hampshire. The State of Liberty and New York City and Philadelphia were included on the agenda. We also went to Gettysburg, the Hershey Chocolate Factory, and all the Washington, DC sites.

We skipped the National Football League Hall of Fame, Major League Baseball Hall of Fame, Basketball Hall of Fame, and the Rock and Roll Hall of Fame. She said I could go back to those places after she was gone, as she had no interest.

The journey ended back home attending a concert by her favorite singer, Kenny Rogers.

The trip was hard for her. She was so glad we made it and appreciated my patience. She knew I was up hours before her. I sat still patiently while she slept and rested. I also sat reading when she did the lymphedema therapy. She always had control of the television remote device in the hotel. I did not turn the TV on when she was resting or asleep.

Tiring of hauling the luggage, medicines, and medical equipment into and out of the hotels happened. I admit that. I couldn't trust the bellhop at the hotels to treat the medical equipment with the tender loving care it needed. The only time I entrusted the machine to hotel staff, I found disconnected hoses and a power cable that had fallen off in the middle of the hallway.

The entire bucket list trip was an adventure in trusting God. What if we had trouble with her chemotherapy medications while 2,500 miles from home? We did, and God cut through the red tape to take care of it.

My attitude, trust in God, and love for my wife somehow allowed me to navigate the journey He had for my loved one and me. He'll do the same for you.

11.2 TRUSTING GOD

Part of caring for a person with a chronic or terminal illness is trusting God. When dealing with a protracted disease, sometimes it is tough to maintain focus or have peace of mind.

The person battling the ailment often dwells on what is happening to them physically, fiscally, and wondering if they'll even have a future. It can be hard.

As a caregiver, you may feel like all you do is manage schedules and provide taxi services. You long for the good old days before the illness took over your life.

Isaiah 26:3 gives us hope as it tells us peace of mind is available. The way to peace is to focus on God, not your problem. It is to trust God. I'll say it again, trust God.

11.3 BIBLE VERSE

Isaiah 26:3 (KJV), "Thou wilt keep him in perfect peace, whose mind is stayed on thee: because he trusteth in thee."

11.4 WHAT THE VERSE MEANS

The key word is trust. We have a requirement to trust God. Trusting in God happens when our mind is focused on Him, not our troubles. It allows us to be kept in God's perfect peace.

11.5 PRAY USING SCRIPTURE

- Heavenly Father, help me keep my mind steadfast on You.
- Thank You for the peace of mind that can only come from God.
- Lord Jesus, help me take my refuge in You.
- God, I know You are the only hope my loved one has in battling her chronic illness.

11.6 RESPONDING TO GOD'S HOPE

1. Name one area where you need to let trust God.
2. Are you thanking God daily for guiding you through the daily challenges? If not, do so now and every day.
3. Are you genuinely trusting God? Ask God to help your unbelief and lack of trust in and for all things.

11.7 TAKEAWAY

The key word is TRUST in God. Trusting in God allows us to be kept in perfect peace.

CHAPTER 12

HOW TO HAVE REAL PROSPERITY

12.1 MY STORY

My wife and I saw the same dermatologist. She is the physician that initially diagnosed Miss Benita's Melanoma Cancer.

Following my wife's initial Melanoma Cancer surgery, I scheduled an appointment to get myself checked. I needed to stay in good health.

At the follow-up appointment, I shared I had a biopsy of a spot in my mouth. The result of the biopsy was oral lichen planus. The oral surgeon referred me to my dermatologist for follow-up treatment.

Oral lichen planus is a chronic inflammatory disease that affects the mucous membrane of the oral cavity.

The dermatologist told me she knew I was under excessive stress with Miss Benita's cancer treatment. She asked if there were additional events happening in my life that were causing me stress.

I shared the added stress I was under from caring for my 89-year-old father. I added it also didn't help that my long-term day job had just completed a significant reduction in force and reorganization. While still employed, I experienced the changes of doing more with less.

She said what I knew. "Stress is everywhere in your life."

Just days before Miss Benita went into hospice care, they diagnosed me with Irritable Bowel Disease. The gastro endocrinologist said while there is no known cause, he was assuming since I had the oral lichen planus and that I was under excessive stress with Miss Benita's cancer treatment that stress was a major contributing factor.

My point is, the stress of caregiving may affect you physically. I do not give medical advice. I do not intend this book as medical advice. If you are having health issues, see your physician for medical advice.

However, for you to provide the best care for your loved one, you need to care for yourself. I saw my physician. She helped me to keep on keeping on and continue to be a caregiver for my spouse.

12.2 REAL PROSPERITY IS IN THE LORD JESUS CHRIST

Part of caring for a person with a chronic or terminal illness realizes our real prosperity is in the Lord Jesus Christ. Today's passage speaks of our mental health and general well-being.

12.3 BIBLE VERSE

3 John 1:2 (KJV), "Beloved, I wish above all things that thou mayest prosper and be in health, even as thy soul prospereth."

12.4 WHAT THE VERSE MEANS

John, the author, is addressing Gaius. John wants Gaius to prosper and have good health equal to his spiritual health.

For your information, in the Book of 3 John, Gaius is John's friend. Gaius was known for his hospitality to travelling preachers, for being faithful and walking in the truth.

12.5 PRAY USING SCRIPTURE

- Heavenly Father, I pray I may prosper and be healthy physically and fiscally. Why? Not to be rich, but to care for my family and pay my medical bills.
- Lord Jesus, I pray I would be in physically good health and that my health would mirror my spiritual health.
- I pray for rest and peace of mind.

12.6 RESPONDING TO GOD'S HOPE

1. Do you have any medical concerns about yourself? List your concerns. Also, seek medical attention for your concerns as soon as possible.
2. Are you getting adequate sleep? If not, talk to your health care professional for advice.
3. Are you eating properly? Seek the help of your health care professional if you have questions.

12.7 TAKEAWAY

Real prosperity is knowing Christ as Savior.

CHAPTER 13

DO NOT LOSE HEART

13.1 MY STORY

It excited my wife when the eleven months of taking the prescription chemotherapy medications ended.

I was expecting her to do a happy dance and to go celebrating her accomplishment. Instead of a time of rejoicing, it became a solemn watershed. She was tired of the handful of pills she took multiple times a day and the way they controlled her life and schedule.

"Jimmie, I will never do chemo again. I know you'll support my decision," she said with the authority and resolve of a drill sergeant barking orders.

Looking at her, I'm sure she saw the questioning, the disappointment, the lack of understanding in my face. I knew better than to question her decision. Her mind was made up. Questioning her decision would bring her to tears. Challenging her choice would breach my commitment to her.

I prayed for God to give me wisdom before I replied. I heard myself say, "You have decided never to do chemo again. You request me to support your decision. Is that correct?"

"Don't be so clinical. Please, do not treat me like you did the children when they were young," she said deliberately with an attitude almost spitting each word at me.

"I'm sorry," I apologized. "I was just restating what you said to make sure I heard you correctly."

"You heard me. Our body isn't made to take these treatments. You can't imagine how horrible they are."

Looking at her, I listened as she continued talking.

"I'm not saying I want to die today. I don't want to die. However, I know that I have an eternity with Jesus Christ in Heaven waiting at the end of this horrible journey. No pain, no suffering, a new body, a grand family reunion with my family and your mother (my mother was deceased, my dad would live another 3 months). It's only because of the ultimate destination that I can continue with this journey with the Melanoma Cancer. Living with cancer is hard. It's terrible."

13.2 NOT LOSING HEART

Part of caring for a person with a chronic illness is not losing heart. Your maintaining a positive attitude helps you to provide the best care. To keep an optimistic view, it is helpful to maintain our outlook from an eternal perspective.

In 2 Corinthians 4:16-18 verse, God is pointing out we should view all earthly adversity in comparison with our future heavenly glory. When we do this, we should be strengthened to endure our human trials.

13.3 BIBLE VERSE

2 Corinthians 4:16-18 (KJV), "For which cause we faint not; but though our outward man perish, yet the inward man is renewed day by day. For our light affliction, which is but for a moment, worketh for us a far more exceeding and eternal weight of glory; While we look not at the things which are seen, but at the things which are not seen: for the things which are seen are temporal; but the things which are not seen are eternal."

13.4 WHAT THE VERSE MEANS

While our bodies (outward man) grow old and suffer from diseases, our spiritual side (inward man) is renewed daily. Too often we only focus on the things we see in this present life. We need to focus on the spiritual, that is the things that are not seen but given to us by God as a future promise.

These are only seen with our "spiritual eyes." It takes belief. A part of faith is believing that what God has promised he will undoubtedly bring to pass. I have confidence in God's word and promises.

13.5 PRAY USING SCRIPTURE

- Heavenly Father, help me focus on You, my loved one's ultimate destination and to never lose heart.
- Lord Jesus, help me remember that while my loved one's outer body is perishing, yet their inward body is being renewed daily.
- God, I realize the chronic illness my loved one is facing won't last forever but is working in them and me a far more exceeding and eternal weight of glory.
- Lord God help me to not look at my loved one's circumstances, which are temporary but to look on the things that are not now seen, but eternal.

13.6 RESPONDING TO GOD'S HOPE

1. Lord Jesus, help me have the courage to see my loved one's situation from their point of view.
2. God in Heaven help me support their choices.
3. Father, help me listen to my loved one.

13.7 TAKEAWAY

It is helpful to maintain our perspective toward our loved one and caregiving from an eternal perspective.

CHAPTER 14

WHERE TO LOOK WHEN YOU ARE SEEKING A SAFE PLACE

14.1 MY STORY

I remember Sunday, December 3, 2017, well. Miss Benita had not been feeling well for the previous two months.

It had started in early October when she worked a week of nights doing a stock reset. She worked retail for the big box store headquartered in Arkansas. I recall her commenting that she rarely minded occasionally working nights.

This time was different. She lacked her usual energy. It was a genuine struggle for her.

We spoke after her first night of work. With a genuine concern, she said the bosses were messing up. Specifically, she mentioned they had printed signs that had left off the last two or three letters of words.

She wasn't happy with my one word response of "really."

She said that when she mentioned it to the manager on duty, he acted as if she was crazy. Even as she insisted something was wrong with the sign, the manager on duty said the signage was okay and ignored her comments. She was told to keep working.

A week later she flew to Denver, Colorado for a week of rest with her two sisters. They met at her older sister's home in the metropolitan Denver area.

Her younger sister flew in from Tennessee to join in the reunion. Miss Benita had made it clear my presence was not needed or wanted for this week. This was to be a special week for her with her sisters.

While in Colorado, my wife got sick. It was her normal nausea, vomiting, and something new, a headache. She went to see a doctor.

The physician told her to take to her nausea medicine and let her doctor know about this spell when she returned home.

Once home, the symptoms lessened. Miss Benita did not see her doctor or call the oncologist. She had a PET scan scheduled in a few days with a follow-up visit to the oncologist, so she would let the doctor know.

She saw the oncologist at the scheduled appointment in early November. The PET Scan was just a full body scan. They did not scan her head.

The body scan did not show any Melanoma Cancer. It only showed the other cancer she had (yes, she had two types of cancer), the neuro-endocrine carcinoid. It had not changed. She mentioned to the doctor the nausea spell on her recent trip to Colorado.

The oncologist commented that while flying and high elevation caused issues in persons with brain tumors, her last brain scans six months earlier had shown no cancer in her head or body. He mentioned if she didn't have the neuro-endocrine carcinoid which had been a cause of her tummy distress for years, he would lean toward the Melanoma Cancer having spread to the brain.

He scheduled a brain scan which after the paperwork, insurance company's initial denial, resubmission, and final approval was ultimately scheduled for the week after Christmas.

By the Friday after Thanksgiving, Miss Benita was having severe nausea issues. As her doctor's office was closed for the holiday, she went to an urgent care facility seeking relief. She passionately declined me taking her to the hospital's emergency room, fearing they would hospitalize her.

The urgent care facility encouraged her to see her primary care doctor on Monday and to call her oncologist to update him.

Miss Benita felt better on Monday. She decided against going to her primary care doctor. "I can't run to her every time I hurt or I would need to move in her office," she said.

She was feeling better when at home by keeping the lights turned off and the windows closed with blackout curtains. Any television or music had to have the volume turned low.

She also mentioned to me that my latest book "Thy Will Be Done: 60 Prayers for the Chronically Ill" wasn't edited very good. She says some sentences aren't complete. It just seems like words are missing, especially at the end of some sentences.

Her words had me remembering her comments on her store signage from early October.

I double checked and the book's editing was fine. Miss Benita became frustrated when I showed her nothing was wrong with the editing.

If I moved the page, the missing words would magically appear for her to read.

I asked if she was having vision problems. She again mentioned the signage at work from back in early October, with letters and words missing.

I suggested we tell this to the managing oncologist and schedule an eye exam. We called and left a message with the oncologist answering service. I also scheduled an eye exam for her later in December.

A few days later on Sunday, December 3, 2018, we attended Sunday morning worship and Bible study. Miss Benita commented that despite the loud music, church is the one place she feels perfectly calm. She added her upset stomach vanishes when in worship services at church. A remarkable peace seems to wrap its arms around her. She feels normal, well, and her heavenly hope engulfs her.

On the afternoon of Thursday, December 7, 2017, Benita called me from the doctor's office parking lot. She had driven herself there from her day job. My help was required to help get her from the car to the doctor's office. She added it has taken her at least ten minutes to get the cell phone to work right where she can call me for help. She was rattled and confused.

I was scared and worried. All my scenes and intuition were screaming this was bad. I dashed to the parking lot, which was just a mile from my house.

She saw the doctor. The physician immediately sends her for an emergency CT Scan of the head. The physician whispers to me she is sure Benita has a brain tumor. She says she will have the scan expedited. She is sure this is terrible.

The CT Scan confirms a large brain tumor.

Miss Benita and I pray. We are next moved to a conference room which allows the CT Scan staff to be with us as we listen on a speakerphone, as the primary care physician explains the results. A staff lady at the CT Scan facility is crying the entire time. The doctor explains the scan showed a brain tumor and we need a category one certified brain trauma facility ASAP. Immediate surgical intervention is required if she is to have a chance of survival.

We go immediately to Presbyterian Hospital in Plano, Texas. It is a certified brain trauma facility.

The surgical neurologist removed a malignant Melanoma Cancer tumor.

The managing oncologist tells me if we had known of the brain tumor Miss Benita shouldn't have flown in October and certainly should not have gone to high elevation in the Rocky Mountains.

The size of her tumor leads him to believe she had it in October and being at elevation caused her sick spell that month while in Colorado. He said in getting records from her primary care doctor helped him get the total picture. Miss Benita had mentioned vision issues just to the primary care physician, not the oncologist.

The oncologist said her flying and going to very high elevation probably caused brain swelling. Being at higher altitude caused her being sick in Colorado. The brain swelling reduced when she was back home at a lower elevation of 595 feet and she felt better.

Well, I could go on and on with what ifs. What ifs lead to regrets. Regrets can lead to despondency and depression. I felt and still feel I let my wife down by not talking to the doctors and making sure they had the total picture.

Please don't go down regret row. You won't enjoy the journey or the destination.

The bottom line is as my spouse's illness worsened it seemed that the only time she was in a state of nirvana was when she was in church, listening to Christian music, or reading or having Scripture read to her. I'm not saying what will work for you or your loved one. I am testifying to the Lord being Miss Benita's stronghold and her place of peace and comfort.

Her experience also shows how difficult diagnosing and treating a disease can be.

. . .

14.2 We Need a Safe Place

Part of caring for a person with a chronic illness realizes that sometimes we need a safe place. We need a place of refuge. A Christian has such a safe place of refuge in God.

The same God who was powerful enough to create the heavens and the Earth and who could destroy the world with the flood in Noah's day is compassionate, kind, and charitable in his nature. He is an unquestionable harbor of protection to those who worship and serve him. He is good. Because of his goodness, He does not ignore or desert the Believer. God accepts, keeps, and preserves the Believers in Jesus Christ.

14.3 BIBLE VERSE

Nahum 1:7 (KJV), "The Lord is good, a stronghold in the day of trouble; and he knoweth them that trust in him."

14.4 WHAT THE VERSE MEANS

But though God is steadfast in His power, yet He is gracious and benevolent in His nature. God is a sure refuge and protection to those who know Him as their Savior, worship Him, serve Him, and put their trust in Him. He knows and pays regard to all such so that they are never neglected by Him. God approves, owns, and preserves us.

14.5 PRAY USING SCRIPTURE

- Heavenly Father, I praise You for Your goodness.
- Thank You for being my stronghold in the day of trouble.
- Thank You for never neglecting me.
- Thank You for Your provision.

14.6 RESPONDING TO GOD'S HOPE

1. Are you going to the Lord God in your day of trouble and every day?
2. Remember to read God's word regularly. There is comfort in God's word. What book of the Bible or passage are you currently reading?
3. Are you treasuring the days you have with your loved one? How? Enjoy the day, whether good or bad, it is the only one you have. Enjoy your loved one.

14.7 TAKEAWAY

God is an unquestionable harbor of protection to those who worship and serve him.

CHAPTER 15

LOVE ME ENOUGH TO LET ME GO

15.1 MY STORY

I still recall the conversation. Rarely have I hated having such a talk. I am forever glad we had the conversation.

"Jimmie, we need to talk," said Miss Benita. I glanced in her direction. While her natural smile and joyous attitude were on her face, it was the tangible seriousness in her voice that caught my attention.

I also realized we needed to talk, RIGHT NOW. Being married to the same person for over forty years helps you understand when she says we need to talk; she means we need to do it NOW.

I didn't take time to get or doing anything. I gave my wife my complete attention.

"What's on your mind," I said as lovingly and supportively as I could. I wanted Miss Benita to know I had her complete attention, and whatever was on her mind was the most critical thing in the world to me. If it was her concern, it was my concern.

"You know I am about to start the radiation treatment on the area of my head where the neurologist removed the brain tumor."

I nodded.

"When the tumor recurs, and it will recur, don't you go letting them cut on my head again. I want no more surgeries. Them cutting on me will not save me. Jesus already saved me when I was a girl."

"So you're saying --" I started.

"I'm saying, love me enough to let me go. It's going to be okay for me. I'll be in heaven with Mama, Daddy, Willie, and Grandma before the hospice people get my time of death called in," she said with a calm and peace of mind that can only come from God.

"Oh, okay," I said suddenly choking out my words.

"Don't go being selfish. Let me go to heaven. Love me enough to let me go. You and the children will be okay. I'll be seeing you all again when you get to heaven. Even the kids that aren't attending church or living for the Lord are going to be there. We trained them up the best we could, we shared Jesus with them, and even when they or you aren't living for the Lord, you're still saved. I know you know that. Like you, they each accepted Christ and knew what they were doing."

I nodded.

Then she quoted from memory Romans 14:8 (KJV), "For whether we live, we live unto the Lord; and whether we die, we die unto the Lord: whether we live, therefore, or die, we are the Lord's."

I teared up.

She added, "Best I can figure, the Lord is leaving you here to write about Him and point others to Him. You need to keep writing religiously. Don't go chasing any Stephen King or Ray Bradbury dreams of fame and fortune. If you honor God, he'll honor you. You know that. You taught me that."

I grabbed a Kleenex.

"The book of devotions you wrote (Prayers for the Chronically Ill) to help me will help others. Write something for those people like you, the ones who are caregivers. You have as hard a job taking care of me and the household as I have been the terminally ill patient. Just keep pointing people to Jesus. We both know Jesus is the only hope anyone has. Now promise me you won't let them cut on me anymore and that you'll write to lead people to Jesus and help Christians grow in their faith."

"I promise," I said as I held her hand and then kissed the back of the hand to seal my pledge.

Eight weeks later, the tumor recurred. At the recurrence, they gave me two options. Option one was surgery, which would extend life a couple of months at the most. Choice two was hospice.

"I need your decision on which option you will choose. I need it now. The operating room is available now and then, not again for several days. Several days will be too late. What do you want to do?" asked the neurological surgeon.

Miss Benita's word reverberated through my head, "Don't go on being selfish. Let me go to heaven. Love me enough to let me go."

"No more surgery. We chose hospice," I said. And then I cried. Loving someone enough to let them die and go to heaven is hard. Loving someone this much also breaks your heart. I know. Making this decision broke my heart. I realized death was at my wife's door.

15.2 WE ARE THE LORD'S

Part of caring for a person with a chronic or terminal illness realizes we are the Lord's.

Today most people live for themselves and live for the moment. This lifestyle differs from how a Christian should live.

The purpose of the Christian life is to do the Lord's will and promote his glory by our life. This doesn't mean you cannot have fun. It allows you to have fun without regrets.

15.3 BIBLE VERSE

Romans 14:8 (KJV), "For whether we live, we live unto the Lord; and whether we die, we die unto the Lord: whether we live, therefore, or die, we are the Lord's."

15.4 WHAT THE VERSE MEANS

The purpose of the Christian life is to do the Lord's will and promote his glory by our life. A Christian should do this because they belong to God. Not only do we belong to God in this life, but we belong to him even as we are dying and after we die.

The passage provides a reminder that the soul does not cease to be conscious at death. We are still the Lord's.

Even when the body is in the grave, we are the Lords. 2 Corinthians 5:8 (KJV) reminds us, "We are confident, I say, and willing rather to be absent from the body, and to be present with the Lord."

15.5 PRAY USING SCRIPTURE

- Heavenly Father, if I live, I live to the Lord. Help me live to the Lord. May You be glorified through my life.
- Lord Jesus, if I die, I die to the Lord. Help me die to the Lord. Help me remember that even in the grave I am Yours.
- I proclaim to the world whether I live or whether I die, I am the Lord's. Thank You, Lord, for the security I have as a Believer in the Lord.

15.6 RESPONDING TO GOD'S HOPE

1. Are you living every day to point people to Jesus? If not, ask God through prayer to help you live for Jesus.
2. Are you reading God's word? Remember, a regular time of reading the Bible will help you as a caregiver. It will strengthen and refresh you spiritually.
3. Who do you know in your loved one's circle of friends that need to know Christ as Savior? Begin praying for God to soften their heart.

15.7 TAKEAWAY

We are the Lords.

CHAPTER 16

HOW TO GIVE YOUR FEARS TO GOD

16.1 MY STORY

My spouse paid the bills each month. Yes, we had a budget and discussed our financial priorities, but she wrote the checks each month and made the electronic payments. We were an old school couple and had a joint checking account.

I had a basic understanding of what bills were due each month but did not know if we paid electronically them or by check. Account numbers, contact information, and other details unknown by me. I was ignorant in these areas.

My spouse clung onto the bill paying. I asked her to tutor or mentor me where I could have some transition if the time came where I had to assume responsibility. She told me if she turned the bill paying over to me she was giving up on life. Bill paying was the last thing she was holding on to do. She held on tight to the financial responsibility.

I pleaded with her to show me her bill paying system. Finally, less than two weeks before she went into hospice care, we talked seriously about finances and bill paying. She started to teach me her system and provide the much needed information to me, but then she just stopped. She said the checkbook is here.

Her next words took me by surprise as she said, "I can't do this. I can't talk to you about the bills. You're a brilliant man and will figure this out. I'm sorry. You'll have to deal with it when the time comes."

I didn't scream or yell. I didn't even roll my eyes. Miss Benita had more confidence in me than I did. I felt scared, helpless. I wondered what I would do and how I would do it when I suddenly had to pay the bills.

A silent prayer crossed my lips. I wish I could tell you it was spiritual, but I asked God why she wouldn't help me. God's still small voice immediately was heard by me. In my mind, I heard LOVE YOUR WIFE. She doesn't need upsetting; she needs to feel my love through you. I'll help you find the answers you need.

Gulp, I turned my fears over to God, trusted him, and to my amazement am still getting it all figured out. All bills have been paid on time. I have developed my routine. Instead of all the worst-case scenarios that ran through my mind. I am surviving.

16.2 GOD'S COMFORT IS AVAILABLE TO YOU

Part of caring for a person with a chronic illness is understanding God's comfort is available for you. He will help you with your fears.

Have you ever been overwhelmed by your thoughts of how you will handle or manage your loved one's chronic illness? Have the "what ifs" overtaken you? Are any of your thoughts confused and even torturing you with the cares and fears about the future?

Psalm 94:19 tells us that God's comfort delights our soul. His promises, contained in His word (the Bible), and the memory of our experiences of His care and kindness to us, afford us comfort. They can restore our discouraged mind.

16.3 BIBLE VERSE

Psalm 94:19 (KJV), "In the multitude of my thoughts within me thy comforts delight my soul."

16.4 WHAT THE VERSE MEANS

When we are fearful because of considering various outcomes and scenarios, listening to non-Biblical counsel from well-meaning friends, or just drowning in self-pity, we need to return to the Lord for proper rest and comfort.

God's comfort satisfies my soul. Focusing and meditating on His Word and teachings comfort me and delight me. True satisfaction only comes from God's Holy Spirit!

Only God can truly remove our fears and give us His perfect peace.

16.5 PRAY USING SCRIPTURE

- Heavenly Father, I confess too often I fill my thoughts with various and confusing ideas. Protect me from the negative thinkers and their contrary counsel.
- Lord Jesus, I admit sometimes being tortured with cares and fears about my future because of my loved one's chronic illness.
- God Almighty, I praise You because Your comfort delights my soul.
- I have heard Your promises taught in Sunday School, heard them preached in church, and have read in the Bible. They comfort me. Your promises remove the fear. Psalm 56:3 (KJV) says, "What time I am afraid, I will trust in thee."
- Lord, the memory of my experiences of Your care and kindness to me, affords me such comfort as they restore my discouraged mind.

16.6 RESPONDING TO GOD'S HOPE

1. Turn your worries and concerns over to God. Take a piece of paper and write five worries you have. When you finish writing your five fears say out loud, God, the concerns I have written I now turn over to you. Crumble the paper and throw it into your trash can.
2. Do not focus on your worries and fears. Instead, thank God that for your ability to provide some care and comfort for your loved one. Remember, sometimes the essential support you provide is being there with them. I call it the ministry of your presence.
3. As I type this, I am praying for the person who is reading these words needs. Know that at least one person has prayed for your needs, cares, and concerns in advance. God ew from the beginning of time that you would have this appointment with caregiving. Maybe that's why I felt impressed to pray for you as I typed this morning.

16.7 TAKEAWAY

"Casting all your care upon him; for he careth for you." 1 Peter 5:7 (KJV)

CHAPTER 17

HOW TO ACCEPT GOD'S HOPE

17. 1 MY STORY

On Thursday, April 2016, I had a surprise in the interoffice mail. The big envelope came with an apology attached on a Post-it Note from the information technology vice president's executive administrative assistant. She expressed her regrets for not getting the dispatch to me sooner.

She shared she had it "for a while, but hadn't gotten it to me with all going on in IT."

In the delivery was a wonderful gift of a necklace for my wife. The gift was from a coworker of mine. It had the word HOPE on it.

Thank you, Cynthia Mitchell, for thinking of my wife, buying, and sending her the necklace. The silver piece of jewelry was beautiful. It put a smile on my sweet wife's face. The necklace with its one-word message was a reminder of the hope through Jesus Christ we all have available.

When we moved my wife into in-patient hospice care, she asked I get the HOPE necklace and put it back on her. She usually wore it all the time, but it was off because of a series of MRIs, CT scans, and PET scans she had during the hospitalization that resulted from the recurrence of her brain tumor.

Cynthia's act of kindness continued to give my wife comfort and hope until her last breath. Cynthia, thank you. You're a beautiful woman inside and out with a caring heart. It blessed me to work with you before I retired. Thanks again.

My wife asked to be buried wearing the necklace. I honored that wish. My wife never lost hope. As death approached, her faith never left. While she would have been glad for a miracle cure of the Melanoma Cancer, she had her hope in Jesus and approached her death with the excitement of a schoolgirl going on a trip to Disney World. She couldn't wait to get on to heaven and to see Jesus. She never mentioned fear, just anticipation.

An interesting side note was when my wife was in in-patient hospice care getting stabilized enough where she could come home for her last days, her registered nurse was named Hope. She had hope with her to the end.

One last thought — A simple act of kindness like a card or a thoughtful gift can touch a person's heart in ways you will never know. If God prompts you to do an act of kindness, please follow through because you may never realize the impact of the hope you're sharing.

17.2 ACCEPTING THE HOPE AVAILABLE THROUGH GOD

Part of caring for a person with a chronic illness is accepting the hope available through God. Everyone needs hope. Job 11:18 tells of the hope we have available in God.

17.3 BIBLE VERSE

Job 11:18 (KJV), "And thou shalt be secure, because there is hope; yea, thou shalt dig about thee, and thou shalt take thy rest in safety."

17.4 WHAT THE VERSE MEANS

Like my wife, you can feel secure because of the hope you have in Jesus Christ. While you will continue to experience life's difficulties, you need not have a gloom and doom or why me Lord attitude.

Your outlook concerning the future should be optimistic because nothing will ultimately be able to harm you or keep your loved one, if they are a Believer in Jesus, from their heavenly destination. You have a firm faith and assurance of your ultimate victory, because of God's love He has shared with You in the Bible's promises which respect the life that now is, and that Heavenly future which for the Christian is the eternal destination.

This knowledge allows you to lie down on the bed and sleep at night in peace and quietness, having nothing to fear.

17.5 PRAY USING SCRIPTURE

- Heavenly Father, we feel secure because there is hope because of You. Help us claim that promise.
- Because of the hope and security that we have in You, we can rest and sleep in peace. Thank You for restful sleep.
- Lord Jesus, help us rest in You.

17.6 RESPONDING TO GOD'S HOPE

1. Do you have hope for the future? I am talking of the hope that's available through knowing Jesus Christ as your Lord and Savior. See Appendix A for information on how to become a Christian.
2. As a caregiver, you'll grow tired and weary. You will have times you doubt you can face another day of taking care of your family member or loved one. Thank God for the hope that you and your charge have through Christ Jesus.

3. Ask God to give you the same level of peace he gave my wife.

17.7 TAKEAWAY

Jesus Christ is the true source of hope.

CHAPTER 18

ACKNOWLEDGE GOD FOR REAL REST

18.1 MY STORY

I had been awake for thirty-three consecutive hours. My marathon of being up began on Tuesday when I had awakened at 5 AM. I had gotten up, checked on my wife, showered and went to Starbucks at 6 AM for my morning writing. From writing, I had headed to the local climate controlled shopping mall where I did my morning walk at 9 AM. Following the exercise, I had an appointment with the dermatologist at 10:30 AM.

I returned home just before lunchtime. I again checked on my wife. She was in her recliner. She said her head was hurting, and she had been trying to call her doctor and me.

Her neurologist had recently reduced her steroids. When the steroids dosage was reduced, she had felt bad, so the doctor increased the dosage to former levels.

Miss Benita assumed this is all that was needed.

Now she couldn't figure out how to use her cell phone. Fear and concern overwhelmed me. I contacted the doctor who changed the medications changed with an immediate doubling of the steroids and sleep overcame her.

Miss Benita did not wake until after 8 PM.

She didn't know me when she awoke. She couldn't tell me what day or month it was.

When I asked if she knew the time she answered "blue?"

We headed for the emergency room at the hospital where only four months earlier she had a brain tumor removed.

I was up all night. My three children took shifts being with me. Around 9 AM on Wednesday morning, the doctor told me the brain tumor had recurred. He said another surgery would only add a few weeks to maybe two months maximum to my sweetie's life. He said your options are surgery or hospice. With hospice, you have days to weeks at best.

Miss Benita and I had previously spoken on what to do if the brain tumor recurred. I followed her wishes and chose hospice. I called my children, my brother, her sisters, my minister, and my best friend informing them of the situation.

The next step was to move her from the intensive care unit to an intermediate care unit where they worked on stabilizing her and helping her regain her faculties. It wasn't until late in the day that they moved her from ICU to a room. My oldest son arrived on the scene. My best friend was there with me as well.

It was nearly noon on Wednesday before I somehow drove home. Instead of sleeping, I prepared the house for my wife's sisters, who were coming in from out of state. I had my sons schedule to shuttle them from the airport to the hospital.

At one-thirty on Wednesday afternoon, I tried to sleep. I slept less than ninety minutes before waking up and returning to the hospital.

When I got back to the hospital, my oldest son and best friend lectured me on the need for rest.

It was late in the day on Wednesday before the massive amount of drugs given my wife took hold and had her where she was conscious, could talk and understand.

I shared with her what was happening. The trust she had in me showed in her eyes and on her face. I still remember her response.

She said with a nervous smile, "I knew the Melanoma Cancer was going to kill me. Just didn't realize it was going to kill me today or in the next few days. Thought I would make survive at least until the end of the year. I hope I live long enough to see Jason (our son) graduate from Southwestern Baptist Theological Seminary in May. Thank you for not letting them cut on me. Thank you for loving me enough to let me go by honoring my wishes."

I nodded.

She squeezed my hand and added, "I've always been in God's hands. He has this. Trust Him. I do."

I went home around 7 PM that evening and cried out to God. Pain and exhaustion overwhelmed me. I remember having Psalm 46:10 come to mind, "Be still and know that I am God…"

Bible verse after Bible verse started filling my mind. I had worked with the children in my church for nearly two decades in a program called "Bible Drill." The program's purpose was Scripture memory. I had memorized the verses along with the children.

Those same verses came to mind, calmed my spirit, and helped me to sleep.

I also was listening to spiritual songs that praised God. The songs calmed my nerves and spirit. I had to slow down enough to experience God's presence.

18.2 SLOW DOWN AND KNOW GOD

Part of caring for a person with a chronic illness is slowing down and knowing God. As we live with the daily challenges of caring for a person with an ongoing disease it is essential, we get adequate rest.

This respite is both physical and spiritual. Psalm 46:10 tells us to slow down, that is to be still and know I am God.

18.3 BIBLE VERSE

Psalm 46:10 (KJV), " Be still, and know that I am God: I will be exalted among the heathen, I will be exalted in the earth."

18.4 WHAT THE VERSE MEANS

Psalm 46:10 is a popular verse for comforting ourselves and others. While the verse encourages the reader to rest and relax in God and reflect on who God is, the verse is actually a wake-up call to be in awe of God.

The verse was written in a time of trouble and war; therefore, we should consider the verse with that context in mind. Back in Psalm 46:1 we were told, "God is our refuge and strength." Psalm 46:10 is telling us to wake up, stop fearing, and acknowledge who our God is. As we care for our loved one, we too should take the time to acknowledge who God is.[1]

18.5 PRAY USING SCRIPTURE

- Heavenly Father, help me be still and know You more intimately, and to feel Your presence.
- Lord Jesus, please help me slow down and even stop when necessary to get to know God.
- I pray I would find rest in the adequacy of God.

18.6 RESPONDING TO GOD'S HOPE

1. Are you getting enough rest? You cannot care for someone twenty-four hours a day, seven days a week. You need help.
2. Are you slowing down where you can hear God and feel his presence?
3. Ask God to help you rest, have the help you need, and to experience his presence.

18.7 TAKEAWAY

We need to take time to acknowledge God. God provides rest for us.

[1] https://www.crosswalk.com/faith/bible-study/what-is-the-meaning-of-the-verse-be-still-and-know-that-i-am-god.html

CHAPTER 19

I'M NOT GOING TO SIT AND WAIT TO DIE

19.1 MY STORY

I'm sure my late wife grew tired of me asking, "What did you weight this morning?"

She would dutifully look at me and then give me the number. It was almost always the same weight. Oh, it may go up or down by a pound or two but generally was the same.

One day she replied, "You're asking my weight to see if cancer is causing me to lose weight. Am I correct?"

Guilty as charged.

Then she schools me. She said, "You're dying like I am. It may not be cancer that's getting you. It's old age. Even though you look a decade younger than your years, Father Time is getting you. The sands that count your days are slipping through the hourglass at an ever-increasing rate — and they'll run out one day."

I nodded.

"I am not going to just sit on the couch and wait to die! There is no way I'm going to sit on the couch wasting away. God still has a purpose for me." She then reminded me she still read her Bible daily, prayed for herself and interceded for others.

She pointed out that God was renewing her inner person daily. Oh, the body was decaying, aging, suffering the ravaging of cancer, but God had her spirit, and inner parson renewed daily.

My wife was smart. I may have had the formal seminary and graduate school education with a couple of fancy masters and a doctoral degree, but she knew so much more from a deeper walk with the Lord in Bible reading, scripture meditation, and time in prayer.

She taught me we shouldn't be obsessed with the physical body. The Christian's faith is far from a fatalistic acceptance of suffering and awaiting death. Every believer in Jesus Christ needs their eyes opened to something else. That something is the continuous restoration of the inner person.

When my late wife was in her last days in hospice care, the incredible calming power of God's word was apparent. I would read from the Book of Psalms in the Bible to her. The occasional anxiousness she had from the terrible pain she suffered would melt away and transform to calm when the words of the Bible were read. Playing favorite hymns and worship songs worked the same miracle. It reminded me of the way she used breathing techniques to mitigate pain when in labor during the delivery of our children. She was so brave. Her tumor was in the brain's area that controlled pain and nausea. Because of the location, normal pain and nausea management medications and techniques did not to work.

I had witnessed Scriptures' calming power on the life of a Believer of Jesus Christ for two-plus decades as a full-time minister working with responsibilities with older adults and pastoral care. Many times, as I would read familiar Bible verses, the chronically or terminally ill person would transform from anxiousness and fear into peacefulness.

Sometimes they even from memory would say or quote the Bible verses with me.

The power of God's word is incredible.

19.2 NOT LOSING HEART

Part of caring for a person with a chronic illness is learning how not to lose heart and help your loved one not develop a gloom and doom attitude. God's word helps you to have a confident acceptance of the reality of life. It enables you to keep the faith.

19.3 BIBLE VERSE

2 Corinthians 4: 16 (KJV), "For which cause we faint not; but though our outward man perish, yet the inward man is renewed day by day."

19.4 WHAT THE VERSE MEANS

Christianity understands the steady decline of the physical body. Though we are rescued from spiritual death and alive with Christ, our bodies remain in the process of decay.

The follower of Christ should recognize that our outer bodies are wasting away. From the moment of birth, we begin to die. It is inescapable unless the Lord Jesus returns first.

The Christian should know increasing inner spiritual strength. God does not forsake his children, but he gives us growing supplies of grace.

The Holy Spirit works in us as an infinite well of life. We are in a constant process of renewal. The Lord does not allow us to be born again and then ignore us. No, He gives us daily spiritual energy.

May we never forget the physical and the spiritual are part of your life every day.

19.5 PRAY USING SCRIPTURE

- Heavenly Father help me to not focus on my decaying or diseased body, but to realize that my inner self is being renewed daily.
- Lord Jesus, help me look to the things that are not seen, not those which are seen.
- God, help me look to the eternal, not the temporal.

19.6 RESPONDING TO GOD'S HOPE

1. Are you spending time in God's word? If not, I encourage you to return to reading your Bible or being reading today for the first time. You can start with just a verse or two. God will speak to you.
2. Are you spending time in prayer? If not, I encourage you to start today. A good beginning would be to pray "God, help me read your Bible. Lord, teach me to pray."
3. Are you obsessed with your loved one's physical appearance? Radiation and chemotherapy take a toll. They may lose their hair. My wife had no hair during her last five months of life. I didn't see her hairless head. I saw her beautiful smile and radiant countenance. She was comfortable without a wig and would wear a chemo beanie when she went to the doctor or on days when she could go out for a walk or meal.

19.7 TAKEAWAY

God's word helps you to have a confident acceptance of the reality of life and enables you to keep the faith.

CHAPTER 20

FAITH FREES ME FROM FEARING DEATH

20.1 MY STORY

As death was imminent for my wife, I did not feel sorry for the brevity of her life. Oh sure, I would have preferred her being healed and having another thirty-plus years with me. After all, dying at sixty-one years old is dying too young.

However, I understood God has our days numbered. From the beginning of time, he knew when you would be born and when you will die.

Psalm 139:16 King James Version (KJV) says, "Thine eyes did see my substance, yet being unperfect; and in thy book all my members were written, which in continuance were fashioned, when as yet there was none of them." In modern English, the verse means that God has ordained or predetermined for me the numbers of days a person will have in their life. He knew when I would be born and knows when I will die. God has this information already written in His book of life.

I found great comfort and security in knowing that God has my life so ordered that I will neither die a day sooner nor live a day longer than what has already been recorded in His book. Life and death decisions are far above my pay grade, so I will happily let Father God take care of that department, thank you very much.

Without a doubt, I know I clearly understand this divine principle. Because of my understanding, I am freed from fearing death. My faith which frees me from this fear allows me to live the life God had designed for me.

Knowing and trusting that God knows best allowed both my wife and me to enjoy the time we had. Instead of weeping over her upcoming death, we could reflect and reminisce. We looked at old pictures, remembering the wonderful, shared events of our family, thankful for our time together.

Miss Benita thanked me for loving her and staying with her until "death do we part." I know it was I who was the real lucky one. Giving thanks to the Lord for our forty-three plus years of marriage was easy. I thank God for the years we had.

When I miss her and feel sad, I focus on the memories, ask God's forgiveness for my failures and regrets, and look forward to the Heavenly reunion I'll have one day with late wife, Miss Benita.

I am thankful for the assurance of Heaven, for the Believer in Jesus Christ.

20.2 THE VALUE OF GIVING THANKS

Part of caring for a person with a chronic illness understands the value of giving thanks for what you have.

When you care for a person with a chronic illness, too often you focus on the negative and the bad. Instead of focusing on the adversity of the situation you are living through, give thanks for what you have.

For the caregiver and their charge who are Believers in Jesus Christ, this includes being thankful knowing that death is not the end. That separation is temporary. You know you will again see each other in Heaven.

20.3 BIBLE VERSE

1 Thessalonians 5:18 (KJV), "In everything give thanks: for this is the will of God in Christ Jesus concerning you."

20.4 WHAT THE VERSE MEANS

The verse reminds us that Christians should not only to pray to God but also give thanks to Him. We should thank him for everything, in every circumstance, in joy and in sorrow.

20.5 PRAY USING SCRIPTURE

- Heavenly Father, help me always show gratitude to family and friends who aid and support us.
- Lord Jesus, help me praise God daily for who He is and for His love and care.
- God Almighty, I thank You for a loving church, Bible fellowship class, our brothers and sisters-in-Christ who help and support me.
- I give thanks for the quality of medical care, and the health insurance that pays for so much of the treatment and prescriptions.

20.6 RESPONDING TO GOD'S HOPE

1. Are you thankful for the days you have with your loved one?
2. Are you grateful for the memories you have? I am amazed God created us with the ability to have remembrances.
3. Have you told your caregiving charge that you're thankful for them and the opportunity to serve them?

20.7 TAKEAWAY

We should thank God for everything, in every circumstance, in joy and in sorrow.

CHAPTER 21

HOW TO LET THE LORD BE YOUR HELPER

21.1 MY STORY

My wife's diagnosis of Melanoma Cancer broke my heart. I promised myself I would be there for her in good times and in the bad times. I would care for her and celebrate every time we received good news. Being there to hold, comfort, and pray for her when the diagnosis was terrible and when she had a bad day was also my job.

My ego initially got in the way as I wanted to prove I was the super best husband ever. I tried to model for the world how to love your wife and care for her.

If I were sincere, I wanted the pat on the back and acclaim of family, coworkers, and friends for being the gold-standard in caregiving. I know I also wanted a well done from Jesus.

After her initial surgery, many people offered help. I took off a couple of weeks from work to care for her. Her sisters flew into town to see how she was doing and help.

All this time I declined more help than I accepted. My Bible fellowship class provided meals and gift cards. They were a blessing.

Over time we settled into the long adjustment to the treatments, a new life normal, and we received fewer offers of help. My stubbornness to accept help continued.

As time passed, I grew weary and had caregiving consuming most of my waking hours. My saying no to offers of help was especially true when Miss Benita had follow-up surgeries. Through this time, I felt guilty when someone else helped. I felt like a failure. It was as if I wasn't doing it all myself that I wasn't being the man or husband I should be.

During her 1001 days after the initial surgery, I was faithful in spending time with the Lord. However, the caregiving took a toll. I developed oral lichen planus, lichen planus, and irritable bowel disease while caring for my spouse. All are autoimmune diseases, and the physicians think stress can contribute to the illnesses. I handled the situation so poorly I made myself sick.

I wonder how much more challenging it would have been if I hadn't spent time with the Lord daily and asked him for his help?

In the last five months of my wife's life, I had someone with me daily helping. I know God touched my wife's sisters' heart to be with her. Family surrounded my wife when she passed away. I was holding my wife's hand and talking with her as she passed into eternity. Her sisters were present. All three of our children were there. Her best girlfriend from high school was present. Only God could have brought all together.

In the last months, I sometimes let the family take my wife to the doctor and radiation treatments from time to time without me. It allowed them to help and see what she was going through. I let her sisters go to the oncologist and hear the reports first hand. Allowing this improved their engagement in caregiving.

21.2 THE LORD IS MY HELPER

Part of caring for a person with a chronic illness is allowing the Lord to be your helper.

When you or our loved one faces a chronic or severe illness, you need the Lord's help as our helper. You also need the courage to face the next hour and the challenges of everyday living. With Christ, you can meet each day without fear.

21.3 BIBLE VERSE

Hebrews 13:6 (KJV), "So that we may boldly say, The Lord is my helper, and I will not fear what man shall do unto me."

21.4 WHAT THE VERSE MEANS

With no hesitation or doubt, in all times of difficulty when we don't know how to pray or how we will make it even through the night, we have an assurance that God will not leave us to suffer.

What can we fear if we have the assurance that the Lord is on our side, and that he will help us?

We fear nothing. Man can do no more to us than God permits, and only what will be for our own good.

We know under whatever trials we may be placed, we need be under no extreme anxiety, for God will be our protector and our friend.

21.5 PRAY USING SCRIPTURE

- Heavenly Father, help us cling to You and keep our total trust in You.
- Lord Jesus, give us the courage to say You are our helper.

- We pray for fear to flee from us. We will not fear what man or disease shall do unto us.

21.6 RESPONDING TO GOD'S HOPE

1. Are you trying to do it all yourself? Be honest.
2. Do your friends and family that have offered to help with the caregiving? List them by name. Consider allowing them to assist.
3. You are not a failure or letting your loved one down if you need to have help. Do you belong to a Bible fellowship class that can help? Maybe there is a ladies Bible study group that would help. How about friends or family? For example, make them aware that you could use someone for sitting with your loved one when you go buy groceries.

21.7 TAKEAWAY

With Christ, you can meet each day without fear.

CHAPTER 22

HOW TO BE COMFORTED DURING TIMES OF HARDSHIPS AND TRIALS

22.1 MY STORY

I thought I knew-how to minister to hurting families and person's facing death. My hubris said I was an expert. After all. I was a seminary trained minister, an ordained minister, and an ordained deacon. I had made thousands of hospital visits, nursing home visits, and been with many persons and their families when death visited. I also had cared for my mother-in-law, and both my parents being the last to see each alive.

It wasn't until I was holding my wife's hand, praying as she took her last breath and hearing the hospice registered nurse pronounce "the time of death was 3:54 PM, April 12, 2018," did I understand the sacrifice in time, emotion, and love that a family member makes in caring for someone they love more than they love themselves.

During the time of my wife's cancer journey, I had with her permission started a Facebook secret group. The group's description was, "A place for those that unconditionally love and care about Benita as she battles Neuroendocrine Carcinoma and Melanoma Cancer. A family of friends, coworkers, and prayer warriors."

As I posted daily updates on her condition, shared how the group members could pray for her, and wrote a short daily devotional thought to encourage both my wife and those praying for her something magical and mystical happened. My wife Benita and I began ministering to those who were praying and ministering to her.

It surprised me when I received the first request for permission to share my daily devotion. The reader asked if it would be okay to copy and send it to a friend that was battling cancer. I had several cousins fighting cancer. A couple of them told me how they looked forward to my posting of the devotion every day. One cousin committed that the short devotional post really ministered to her because she knew we were living what she was experiencing. This was a real first person experience and prayer instead of just words on a page.

It was with her words that I realized how God was using the bad in our life for good to others. My wife Benita would write and send cards to others until about ten days before she died. She would share encouragement and how God was sustaining her during her cancer experience. She could comfort others despite her tribulation.

22.2 DEVELOPING COMPASSION FOR OTHERS

Part of caring for a person with a chronic illness is developing compassion for others. Caring for a person with a long-lasting disease affects people in different ways. Depression may come to live with some people. Other persons can become bitter. Withdrawal from friends and family can occur with some. You will find yourself tired, more tired than you thought you could ever become.

For the Believer in Jesus Christ, the chronic illness often mellows our heart to make us more compassionate. The persistent disease allows us empathy. It often becomes the point of rapport where we can care for and minister to not only our loved one but others now walking down the pathway we have recently or are currently helping our loved navigate.

22.3 TODAY'S BIBLE VERSES

2 Corinthians 1:3-4 (KJV), "Blessed be God, even the Father of our Lord Jesus Christ, the Father of mercies, and the God of all comfort; Who comforted us in all our tribulation, that we may be able to comfort them which are in any trouble, by the comfort wherewith we ourselves are comforted of God."

22.4 WHAT THE VERSES MEAN

The verses are a reminder of what a wonderful God we have. He is the one who comforts and strengthens us in our hardships and trials.

Why does He do this? He does this where we can help others.

When family, friends, or coworkers are troubled, needing our support, sympathy, and encouragement, we can pass on to them the help and comfort God has given us.

22.5 PRAY USING SCRIPTURE

- Heavenly Father, I praise You for how wonderful you are.
- I acknowledge You are the Father of the Lord Jesus.
- I proclaim You as the one who wonderfully comforts and strengthens me in hardships and trials.
- Thank you for teaching me how to soothe others by your example to me where I can give sympathy and encouragement.

22.6 RESPONDING TO GOD'S HOPE

1. Who do you know that could use a word of support today?
2. How can you prove that supportive word? A card, a phone call, an email or text?

3. Name two things you learned in your journey as a caregiver that help you comfort others.

22.7 TAKEAWAY

As a caregiver we can pass on to others the help and comfort God has given us.

CHAPTER 23

HOW TO HANG ON

23.1 MY STORY

The date was April 11, 2018. The day of the week was a Wednesday. I woke up at the usual time of 5 AM. Stepping into the master bedroom where my wife was resting, I took her hand and held it. Leaning over the hospital bed, I kissed her forehead. Then I said, I love you. She squeezed my hand, and her lips moved, mouthing I love you. I softly kissed her lips. I could feel their warmth and her returning the kiss.

We were blessed with a critical care registered nurse in our home twenty-four hours a day. Looking at the nurse, I said I was going to Starbucks for a couple of hours to have morning coffee and write. Telling her I would be back home by 8 AM, I then reminded her two of my adult children, and my wife's sisters were in the house if needed. I would only be ten to fifteen minutes away. My contact information was on a paper I handed the nurse.

I then read Psalm 23 to my wife, prayed with her, and feed her a container of flavored shaved ice before I stole another kiss and then headed to Starbucks. As I drove to the coffeehouse, my heart was heavy. Death was near.

Around 7:30 AM I had a telephone call from the hospice supervising nurse. She was at my house checking on the situation. She had arrived at the shift change to speak to the overnight nurse and brief the incoming nurse. The message, death was imminent. She encouraged me to get home as soon as possible to say any last goodbyes.

Miss Benita and I had already said our goodbyes. I never left her side without saying a last farewell, just in case she died when I wasn't there. I wanted to be present with her, holding her hand when the time came for her to depart to heaven, so I hastily retreated to my house.

When I arrived, I could see a marked change in my wife. In only two hours she had moved much closer to death's doorway.

No, she didn't die on April 11. Benita Kepler passed away at 3:54 pm on April 12, 2018. I wrote that day, "She is in Jesus' loving arms in heaven. Her husband, children, sisters, and friends surrounded her when she went to be with Jesus in heaven."

23.2 HANG ON

Part of caring for a person with a chronic illness understands the value of hanging on to God.

You will get to the point in caregiving that only with God's help can you make it through the next few minutes or day. You will find yourself exhausted mentally, physically, and spiritually.

All you can do is grab hold of and hang on to God. Holding on to God allows you to finish strong.

23.3 BIBLE VERSE

2 Corinthians 4:8-9 (KJV), "We are troubled on every side, yet not distressed; we are perplexed, but not in despair; Persecuted, but not forsaken; cast down, but not destroyed;"

23.4 WHAT THE VERSE MEANS

The best commentary on the Bible is the Bible itself. Here are Biblical principles that explain the verse. These seven principles give the Biblical alternative of how to hang on when you feel you're at the end of your rope.

Principle One: I must not forget God loves me. Don't lose heart!

2 Corinthians 4:1 (KJV), "Therefore seeing we have this ministry, as we have received mercy, we faint not;"

1 Corinthians 15:10 (KJV), "But by the grace of God I am what I am: and his grace which was bestowed upon me was not in vain; but I labored more abundantly than they all: yet not I, but the grace of God which was with me."

It's not who we are. It's whose we are!

Remember, our performance does not give us our worth. God's grace provides us with the power to start over.

Romans 8:37 (KJV), "Nay, in all these things we are more than conquerors through him that loved us."

Principle Two: I must keep a clear conscience.

2 Corinthians 4:2 (KJV), "But have renounced the hidden things of dishonesty, not walking in craftiness, nor handling the word of God

deceitfully; but by manifestation of the truth commending ourselves to every man's conscience in the sight of God."

We must have integrity. We must have character.

Principle Three: It is not about me.

2 Corinthians 4:5 (KJV), "For we preach not ourselves, but Christ Jesus the Lord; and ourselves your servants for Jesus' sake."

Your ego will only take you so far.

Principle Four: I cannot do it all.

2 Corinthians 4:7 (KJV), "But we have this treasure in earthen vessels, that the excellency of the power may be of God, and not of us."

We must pace ourselves. Life is a journey, not a sprint.

Principle Five: Love, love, love.

2 Corinthians 4:15 (KJV), "For all things are for your sakes, that the abundant grace might through the thanksgiving of many redound to the glory of God."

Principle Six: Take time to refresh, renew, and revive.

2 Corinthians 4:16 (KJV), "For which cause we faint not; but though our outward man perish, yet the inward man is renewed day by day."

. . .

Principle Seven: I must keep my eye on the goal.

2 Corinthians 4:17-18 (KJV), "For our light affliction, which is but for a moment, worketh for us a far more exceeding and eternal weight of glory; While we look not at the things which are seen, but at the things which are not seen: for the things which are seen are temporal; but the things which are not seen are eternal."

Remember, you cannot do your best at caregiving if you do not face your troubles and hang on until you reach your goal.

23.5 PRAY USING SCRIPTURE

- Heavenly Father, help me cling to You.
- Lord Jesus, help me ask Your help daily as I keep on keeping on.
- God Almighty, help my eyes to be fixed on the unseen.

23.6 RESPONDING TO GOD'S HOPE

1. Do you remember God loves you?
2. Is your conscience clear? Maybe you feel bitter about having to care for your loved ones. If so, ask God's forgiveness.
3. Are you seeking God's help and guidance? Ask God for his help.

23.7 TAKEAWAY

Holding on to God allows you to finish strong.

APPENDIX A

HOW TO BECOME A CHRISTIAN

Being a good person doesn't get you to heaven. Being saved or born-again does. Here's my story of how I accepted Jesus Christ and became a Christian.

On July 11, 1977, my life changed. If you look up that date in history, you will find nothing historically significant happened on that Sunday. It was a remarkable day for me. Sunday, July 11, 1977, was the watershed event in my life.

While attending First Baptist Church of Lakewood in Tacoma, Washington, I noticed a group of men that seemed to have what I was missing. I attended a Bible study with them.

Here I found God has given us an essential manual for life. The manual is the Bible. God has the answers to the problems and emptiness we may face. I found out I was here for a purpose, and not by accident. I learned Jesus loves me and desires to have a personal relationship with me. However, sin separated me from Him.

A.1 I REALIZED I HAD A SIN PROBLEM

The Bible says in Romans 3:23 (KJV), "For all have sinned and fall short of the glory of God."

But no one is perfect! We have all sinned and therefore cannot save ourselves by just living a good life.

Why not?

A.2 I LEARNED THERE WAS A PENALTY TO BE PAID FOR MY SIN

The Bible says in Romans 6:23 (KJV), "For the wages of sin is death; but the gift of God is eternal life through Jesus Christ our Lord."

A.3 I LEARNED GOD GIVES US A PROMISE

The Bible says in John 3:16 (KJV), "For God so loved the world, that he gave his only begotten Son, that whosoever believeth in him shall not perish, but have everlasting life."

A.4 I LEARNED GOD MADE A PROVISION FOR ME

The Bible says in Romans 10:9-10, 13 (KJV), "That if thou shalt confess with thy mouth the Lord Jesus, and shalt believe in thine heart that God hath raised him from the dead, thou shalt be saved. For with the heart man believeth unto righteousness; and with the mouth confession is made unto salvation. For whosoever shall call upon the name of the Lord shall be saved."

A.5 I PRAYED TO ACCEPT THE GIFT OF ETERNAL LIFE THROUGH JESUS

I prayed, "Jesus, I know I am a sinner. I believe You died for my sins and rose from the grave so that I might have eternal life in Heaven with

You. I willingly repent of my sins and ask you to come into my heart and life. Take control of my words, thoughts, and actions. I place all of my trust in You for my salvation. I accept You as my Lord and Savior, and this free gift of eternal life. Amen."

Since then, my life has not been perfect. It's been far from it. I've messed up from time to time, sometimes failing miserably in my decisions and choices. However, I have had direction and purpose in my life. I know where I am headed. I have the Bible to give me the principles for daily living. I am never alone. I have had real peace for the last 40 plus years.

How about you? Have you ever been saved?

A.6 YOU CAN DO LIKE I DID

Romans 10:9-10, 13 tells us, "That if thou shalt confess with thy mouth the Lord Jesus, and shalt believe in thine heart that God hath raised him from the dead, thou shalt be saved. For with the heart man believeth unto righteousness, and with the mouth confession is made unto salvation. ... For whosoever shall call upon the name of the Lord shall be saved."

Why Not Pray This Simple Prayer and Accept Jesus Christ Today?

APPENDIX B

TWENTY-ONE BIBLE VERSES THAT TEACH US TO WAIT UPON THE LORD

B.1 WAIT UPON THE LORD

The Bible is full of verses that remind us to wait on the Lord.

Have you ever read in the Bible the phrase "wait upon the Lord" and wondered what it means? Those four words have two basic meanings in the Bible.

B.2 OLD TESTAMENT MEANING

When "wait upon the Lord" is used in the Old Testament, the Nation of Israel, the people of God, and individual people were told to wait on God's providential care.

B.3 NEW TESTAMENT MEANING

Often when the phrase "wait upon the Lord" is used in the New Testament it refers to Jesus' second coming.

An ordinary meaning in most all biblical instances for waiting on the Lord is having the expectant trust and hope in God's movement and activity.

B.4 TWENTY-ONE BIBLE VERSES THAT ADVISE US TO WAIT UPON THE LORD:

1. Psalm 27:14 (KJV), "Wait on the Lord: be of good courage, and he shall strengthen thine heart: wait, I say, on the Lord."
2. Psalm 25:3 (KJV), "Yea, let none that wait on thee be ashamed: let them be ashamed which transgress without cause."
3. Psalm 25:5 (KJV), "Lead me in thy truth, and teach me: for thou art the God of my salvation; on thee do I wait all the day."
4. Psalm 37:9 (KJV), "For evildoers shall be cut off: but those that wait upon the Lord, they shall inherit the earth."
5. Psalm 62:5 (KJV), "My soul, wait thou only upon God; for my expectation is from him."
6. Psalm 69:3 (KJV), "I am weary of my crying: my throat is dried: mine eyes fail while I wait for my God."
7. Psalm 123:2 (KJV), "Behold, as the eyes of servants look unto the hand of their masters, and as the eyes of a maiden unto the hand of her mistress; so our eyes wait upon the Lord our God, until that he have mercy upon us."
8. Isaiah 40:31 (KJV), "But they that wait upon the Lord shall renew their strength; they shall mount up with wings as eagles; they shall run, and not be weary; and they shall walk, and not faint."
9. Isaiah 8:17 (KJV), "And I will wait upon the Lord, that hideth his face from the house of Jacob, and I will look for him."
10. Jeremiah 14:22 (KJV), "Are there any among the vanities of the Gentiles that can cause rain? or can the heavens give

showers? art not thou he, O Lord our God? therefore we will wait upon thee: for thou hast made all these things."
11. Mark 15:43 (KJV), "Joseph of Arimathaea, an honourable counseller, which also waited for the kingdom of God, came, and went in boldly unto Pilate, and craved the body of Jesus."
12. Luke 2:25 (KJV), "And, behold, there was a man in Jerusalem, whose name was Simeon; and the same man was just and devout, waiting for the consolation of Israel: and the Holy Ghost was upon him."
13. Luke 12:35-40 (KJV), "Let your loins be girded about, and your lights burning; And ye yourselves like unto men that wait for their lord, when he will return from the wedding; that when he cometh and knocketh, they may open unto him immediately. Blessed are those servants, whom the lord when he cometh shall find watching: verily I say unto you, that he shall gird himself, and make them to sit down to meat, and will come forth and serve them."
14. Romans 8:23-25 (KJV), "And not only they, but ourselves also, which have the first fruits of the Spirit, even we ourselves groan within ourselves, waiting for the adoption, to wit, the redemption of our body. For we are saved by hope: but hope that is seen is not hope: for what a man seeth, why doth he yet hope for? But if we hope for that we see not, then do we with patience wait for it."
15. 1 Corinthians 1:7 (KJV), "So that ye come behind in no gift; waiting for the coming of our Lord Jesus Christ:"
16. 1 Corinthians 4:5 (KJV), "Therefore judge nothing before the time, until the Lord come, who both will bring to light the hidden things of darkness, and will make manifest the counsels of the hearts: and then shall every man have praise of God."
17. Galatians 5:5 (KJV), "For we through the Spirit wait for the hope of righteousness by faith."
18. Titus 2:13 (KJV), "Looking for that blessed hope, and the

glorious appearing of the great God and our Saviour Jesus Christ;"
19. Hebrews 9:28 (KJV) "So Christ was once offered to bear the sins of many; and unto them that look for him shall he appear the second time without sin unto salvation."
20. James 5:7-8 (KJV), "Be patient therefore, brethren, unto the coming of the Lord. Behold, the husbandman waiteth for the precious fruit of the earth, and hath long patience for it, until he receive the early and latter rain. Be ye also patient; stablish your hearts: for the coming of the Lord draweth nigh."
21. Revelation 6:9-11 (KJV), "And when he had opened the fifth seal, I saw under the altar the souls of them that were slain for the word of God, and for the testimony which they held: And they cried with a loud voice, saying, How long, O Lord, holy and true, dost thou not judge and avenge our blood on them that dwell on the earth? And white robes were given unto every one of them; and it was said unto them, that they should rest yet for a little season, until their fellow servants also and their brethren, that should be killed as they were, should be fulfilled."

APPENDIX C

TWENTY BIBLE VERSES TO HELP WITH WORRY AND ANXIETY

1. Joshua 10:25 (KJV), "And Joshua said unto them, Fear not, nor be dismayed, be strong and of good courage: for thus shall the Lord do to all your enemies against whom ye fight."
2. Ruth 1:12 (KJV), "Turn again, my daughters, go your way; for I am too old to have an husband. If I should say, I have hope, if I should have an husband also to night, and should also bear sons;"
3. Psalm 3:2-6 (KJV), "Many there be which say of my soul, There is no help for him in God. Selah. But thou, O LORD, art a shield for me; my glory, and the lifter up of mine head. I cried unto the LORD with my voice, and he heard me out of his holy hill. Selah. I laid me down and slept; I awaked; for the LORD sustained me. I will not be afraid of ten thousands of people, that have set themselves against me round about."
4. Psalm 147:11 (KJV), "The Lord taketh pleasure in them that fear him, in those that hope in his mercy."
5. Proverbs 13:12 (KJV), "Hope deferred maketh the heart sick: but when the desire cometh, it is a tree of life."
6. Isaiah 40:31 (KJV), "But they that wait upon the LORD shall renew their strength; they shall mount up with wings as

eagles; they shall run, and not be weary; and they shall walk, and not faint."
7. Jeremiah 29:11 (KJV), "For I know the thoughts that I think toward you, saith the LORD, thoughts of peace, and not of evil, to give you an expected end."
8. Romans 5:2-7 (KJV), "By whom also we have access by faith into this grace wherein we stand, and rejoice in hope of the glory of God. And not only so, but we glory in tribulations also: knowing that tribulation worketh patience; And patience, experience; and experience, hope: And hope maketh not ashamed; because the love of God is shed abroad in our hearts by the Holy Ghost which is given unto us. For when we were yet without strength, in due time Christ died for the ungodly. For scarcely for a righteous man will one die: yet peradventure for a good man some would even dare to die."
9. Romans 5:5 (KJV), "And hope does not put us to shame, because God's love has been poured out into our hearts through the Holy Spirit, who has been given to us."
10. Romans 8:24-25 (KJV), "For we are saved by hope: but hope that is seen is not hope: for what a man seeth, why doth he yet hope for? But if we hope for that we see not, then do we with patience wait for it."
11. Romans 8:28-29 (KJV), "And we know that all things work together for good to them that love God, to them who are the called according to his purpose. For whom he did foreknow, he also did predestinate to be conformed to the image of his Son, that he might be the firstborn among many brethren."
12. Romans 15:13 (KJV), "May the God of hope fill you with all joy and peace as you trust in him, so that you may overflow with hope by the power of the Holy Spirit."
13. 1 Corinthians 15:54-58 (KJV), "So when this corruptible shall have put on incorruption, and this mortal shall have put on immortality, then shall be brought to pass the saying that is written, Death is swallowed up in victory. O death, where is thy sting? O grave, where is thy victory? The sting of death is

sin; and the strength of sin is the law. But thanks be to God, which giveth us the victory through our Lord Jesus Christ. Therefore, my beloved brethren, be ye stedfast, unmoveable, always abounding in the work of the Lord, forasmuch as ye know that your labour is not in vain in the Lord."
14. Galatians 6:8 (KJV), "For he that soweth to his flesh shall of the flesh reap corruption; but he that soweth to the Spirit shall of the Spirit reap life everlasting."
15. Philippians 1:6 (KJV), "Being confident of this very thing, that he which hath begun a good work in you will perform it until the day of Jesus Christ:"
16. Philippians 3:13-14 (KJV), "Brethren, I count not myself to have apprehended: but this one thing I do, forgetting those things which are behind, and reaching forth unto those things which are before, I press toward the mark for the prize of the high calling of God in Christ Jesus."
17. Colossians 1:27 (KJV), "To whom God would make known what is the riches of the glory of this mystery among the Gentiles; which is Christ in you, the hope of glory:"
18. Colossians 3:1-2 (KJV), "If ye then be risen with Christ, seek those things which are above, where Christ sitteth on the right hand of God. Set your affection on things above, not on things on the earth."
19. 1 Peter 5:10 (KJV), "But the God of all grace, who hath called us unto his eternal glory by Christ Jesus, after that ye have suffered a while, make you perfect, stablish, strengthen, settle you."
20. Hebrew 11:11 (KJV), "Through faith also Sara herself received strength to conceive seed, and was delivered of a child when she was past age, because she judged him faithful who had promised."

APPENDIX D

TAKEAWAYS

TAKEAWAY FROM CHAPTER 1

Part of caring for a person with a chronic illness understands that fear of the unknown and fear of the journey is normal.

TAKEAWAY FROM CHAPTER 2

Part of learning to care for a person with a chronic illness understands how to rely on the Lord.

TAKEAWAY FROM CHAPTER 3

God gives you permission to cry. Your Heavenly Father even collects your tears in a bottle.

TAKEAWAY FROM CHAPTER 4

God goes with us both sustaining and provides the rest we need.

TAKEAWAY FROM CHAPTER 5

During our life we face many challenges. With Jesus, we can face each day.

TAKEAWAY FROM CHAPTER 6

We need to spend time with God. We do this by reading the Bible, listening to Hymns and spiritual songs, listening to sermons, and by prayer and meditation. Spending time with God helps us make Godly decisions and helps us to wait upon the Lord and His timing.

TAKEAWAY FROM CHAPTER 7

Having a positive attitude helps as you care for your loved one. It helps both you and your loved one.

TAKEAWAY FROM CHAPTER 8

The Bible teaches God has numbered our days. We need to live each day to the fullest.

TAKEAWAY FROM CHAPTER 9

Real peace comes from God.

TAKEAWAY FROM CHAPTER 10

God's Word is perfect. His Word provides direction for your life.

TAKEAWAY FROM CHAPTER 11

The key word is TRUST in God. Trusting in God allows us to be kept in perfect peace.

CAREGIVING

TAKEAWAY FROM CHAPTER 12

Real prosperity is knowing Christ as Savior.

TAKEAWAY FROM CHAPTER 13

It is helpful to maintain our perspective toward our loved one and caregiving from an eternal perspective.

TAKEAWAY FROM CHAPTER 14

God is an unquestionable harbor of protection to those who worship and serve him.

TAKEAWAY FROM CHAPTER 15

We are the Lords.

TAKEAWAY FROM CHAPTER 16

"Casting all your care upon him; for he careth for you." 1 Peter 5:7 (KJV)

TAKEAWAY FROM CHAPTER 17

Jesus Christ is the true source of hope.

TAKEAWAY FROM CHAPTER 18

We need to take time to acknowledge God. God provides rest for us.

TAKEAWAY FROM CHAPTER 19

God's word helps you to have a confident acceptance of the reality of life and enables you to keep the faith.

TAKEAWAY FROM CHAPTER 20

We should thank God for everything, in every circumstance, in joy and in sorrow.

TAKEAWAY FROM CHAPTER 21

With Christ, you can meet each day without fear.

TAKEAWAY FROM CHAPTER 22

As a caregiver we can pass on to others the help and comfort God has given us.

TAKEAWAY FROM CHAPTER 23

Holding on to God allows you to finish strong.

APPENDIX E

BIBLE VERSE INDEX

1. Exodus 33:14 (KJV), "My presence will go with you, and I will give you rest."
2. Deuteronomy 31:6 (KJV), "Be strong and of a good courage, fear not, nor be afraid of them: for the Lord thy God, he it is that doth go with thee; he will not fail thee, nor forsake thee."
3. Joshua 10:25 (KJV), "And Joshua said unto them, Fear not, nor be dismayed, be strong and of good courage: for thus shall the Lord do to all your enemies against whom ye fight."
4. Ruth 1:12 (KJV), "Turn again, my daughters, go your way; for I am too old to have an husband. If I should say, I have hope, if I should have an husband also to night, and should also bear sons;"
5. Job 11:18 (KJV), "And thou shalt be secure, because there is hope; yea, thou shalt dig about thee, and thou shalt take thy rest in safety."
6. Job 14:5 (KJV), "Seeing his days are determined, the number of his months are with thee, thou hast appointed his bounds that he cannot pass;"
7. Job 14:5-7 (KJV), "Seeing his days are determined, the number of his months are with thee, thou hast appointed his

bounds that he cannot pass; Turn from him, that he may rest, till he shall accomplish, as an hireling, his day."
8. Job 21:21 (KJV), "For what does he care for his household after him, When the number of his months is cut off?
9. Psalm 3:2-6 (KJV), "Many there be which say of my soul, There is no help for him in God. Selah. But thou, O LORD, art a shield for me; my glory, and the lifter up of mine head. I cried unto the LORD with my voice, and he heard me out of his holy hill. Selah. I laid me down and slept; I awaked; for the LORD sustained me. I will not be afraid of ten thousands of people, that have set themselves against me round about."
10. Psalm 25:3 (KJV), "Yea, let none that wait on thee be ashamed: let them be ashamed which transgress without cause."
11. Psalm 25:5 (KJV), "Lead me in thy truth, and teach me: for thou art the God of my salvation; on thee do I wait all the day."
12. Psalm 27:14 (KJV), "Wait on the Lord: be of good courage, and he shall strengthen thine heart: wait, I say, on the Lord."
13. Psalm 31:15 (KJV), "My times are in Your hand; Deliver me from the hand of my enemies and from those who persecute me."
14. Psalm 34:19, (KJV) "Many are the afflictions of the righteous, but the Lord delivers him out of them all."
15. Psalm 37:9 (KJV), "For evildoers shall be cut off: but those that wait upon the Lord, they shall inherit the earth."
16. Psalm 39:4 (KJV), "Lord, make me to know mine end, and the measure of my days, what it is: that I may know how frail I am."
17. Psalm 46:10 (KJV), " Be still, and know that I am God: I will be exalted among the heathen, I will be exalted in the earth."
18. Psalm 56:8-9 (KJV), "Thou tellest my wanderings: put thou my tears into thy bottle: are they not in thy book? When I cry unto thee, then shall mine enemies turn back: this I know; for God is for me."

19. Psalm 62:5 (KJV), "My soul, wait thou only upon God; for my expectation is from him."
20. Psalm 69:3 (KJV), "I am weary of my crying: my throat is dried: mine eyes fail while I wait for my God."
21. Psalm 94:19 (KJV), "In the multitude of my thoughts within me thy comforts delight my soul."
22. Psalm 123:2 (KJV), "Behold, as the eyes of servants look unto the hand of their masters, and as the eyes of a maiden unto the hand of her mistress; so our eyes wait upon the Lord our God, until that he have mercy upon us."
23. Psalm 139:16 (KJV), "Thine eyes did see my substance, yet being unperfect; and in thy book all my members were written, which in continuance were fashioned, when as yet there was none of them."
24. Psalm 143:8 (KJV), "Cause me to hear thy lovingkindness in the morning; for in thee do I trust: cause me to know the way wherein I should walk; for I lift up my soul unto thee."
25. Psalm 147:11 (KJV), "The Lord taketh pleasure in them that fear him, in those that hope in his mercy."
26. Proverbs 13:12 (KJV), "Hope deferred maketh the heart sick: but when the desire cometh, it is a tree of life."
27. Proverbs 17:22 (KJV), "A merry heart doeth good like a medicine: but a broken spirit drieth the bones."
28. Ecclesiastes 3:2 (KJV), "A time to give birth and a time to die; A time to plant and a time to uproot what is planted."
29. Isaiah 8:17 (KJV), "And I will wait upon the Lord, that hideth his face from the house of Jacob, and I will look for him."
30. Isaiah 26:3 (KJV), "Thou wilt keep him in perfect peace, whose mind is stayed on thee: because he trusteth in thee."
31. Isaiah 40:31 (KJV), "But they that wait upon the Lord shall renew their strength; they shall mount up with wings as eagles; they shall run, and not be weary; and they shall walk, and not faint."
32. Jeremiah 14:22 (KJV), "Are there any among the vanities of the Gentiles that can cause rain? or can the heavens give

showers? art not thou he, O Lord our God? therefore we will wait upon thee: for thou hast made all these things."
33. Jeremiah 15:16 (KJV), "Thy words were found, and I did eat them; and thy word was unto me the joy and rejoicing of mine heart: for I am called by thy name, O Lord God of hosts."
34. Jeremiah 29:11 (KJV), "For I know the thoughts that I think toward you, saith the LORD, thoughts of peace, and not of evil, to give you an expected end."
35. Nahum 1:7 (KJV), "The Lord is good, a stronghold in the day of trouble; and he knoweth them that trust in him."
36. Mark 15:43 (KJV), "Joseph of Arimathaea, an honourable counseller, which also waited for the kingdom of God, came, and went in boldly unto Pilate, and craved the body of Jesus."
37. Luke 2:25 (KJV), "And, behold, there was a man in Jerusalem, whose name was Simeon; and the same man was just and devout, waiting for the consolation of Israel: and the Holy Ghost was upon him."
38. Luke 12:35-40 (KJV), "Let your loins be girded about, and your lights burning; And ye yourselves like unto men that wait for their lord, when he will return from the wedding; that when he cometh and knocketh, they may open unto him immediately. Blessed are those servants, whom the lord when he cometh shall find watching: verily I say unto you, that he shall gird himself, and make them to sit down to meat, and will come forth and serve them."
39. John 3:16 (KJV), "For God so loved the world, that he gave his only begotten Son, that whosoever believeth in him shall not perish, but have everlasting life."
40. John 14:27 (KJV), "Peace I leave with you, my peace I give unto you: not as the world giveth, give I unto you. Let not your heart be troubled, neither let it be afraid."
41. Romans 3:23 (KJV), "For all have sinned and fall short of the glory of God."
42. Romans 5:2-7 (KJV), "By whom also we have access by faith into this grace wherein we stand, and rejoice in hope of the

glory of God. And not only so, but we glory in tribulations also: knowing that tribulation worketh patience; And patience, experience; and experience, hope: And hope maketh not ashamed; because the love of God is shed abroad in our hearts by the Holy Ghost which is given unto us. For when we were yet without strength, in due time Christ died for the ungodly. For scarcely for a righteous man will one die: yet peradventure for a good man some would even dare to die."

43. Romans 5:5 (KJV), "And hope does not put us to shame, because God's love has been poured out into our hearts through the Holy Spirit, who has been given to us."
44. Romans 6:23 (KJV), "For the wages of sin is death; but the gift of God is eternal life through Jesus Christ our Lord."
45. Romans 8:23-25 (KJV), "And not only they, but ourselves also, which have the first fruits of the Spirit, even we ourselves groan within ourselves, waiting for the adoption, to wit, the redemption of our body. For we are saved by hope: but hope that is seen is not hope: for what a man seeth, why doth he yet hope for? But if we hope for that we see not, then do we with patience wait for it."
46. Romans 8:24-25 (KJV), "For we are saved by hope: but hope that is seen is not hope: for what a man seeth, why doth he yet hope for? But if we hope for that we see not, then do we with patience wait for it."
47. Romans 8:28-29 (KJV), "And we know that all things work together for good to them that love God, to them who are the called according to his purpose. For whom he did foreknow, he also did predestinate to be conformed to the image of his Son, that he might be the firstborn among many brethren."
48. Romans 8:37 (KJV), "Nay, in all these things we are more than conquerors through him that loved us."
49. Romans 10:9-10, 13 (KJV), "That if thou shalt confess with thy mouth the Lord Jesus, and shalt believe in thine heart that God hath raised him from the dead, thou shalt be saved. For with the heart man believeth unto righteousness; and with the

mouth confession is made unto salvation. For whosoever shall call upon the name of the Lord shall be saved."

50. Romans 14:8 (KJV), "For whether we live, we live unto the Lord; and whether we die, we die unto the Lord: whether we live therefore, or die, we are the Lord's."
51. Romans 15:13 (KJV), "May the God of hope fill you with all joy and peace as you trust in him, so that you may overflow with hope by the power of the Holy Spirit."
52. 1 Corinthians 1:7 (KJV), "So that ye come behind in no gift; waiting for the coming of our Lord Jesus Christ:"
53. 1 Corinthians 4:5 (KJV), "Therefore judge nothing before the time, until the Lord come, who both will bring to light the hidden things of darkness, and will make manifest the counsels of the hearts: and then shall every man have praise of God."
54. 1 Corinthians 15:10 (KJV), "But by the grace of God I am what I am: and his grace which was bestowed upon me was not in vain; but I labored more abundantly than they all: yet not I, but the grace of God which was with me."
55. 1 Corinthians 15:54-58 (KJV), "So when this corruptible shall have put on incorruption, and this mortal shall have put on immortality, then shall be brought to pass the saying that is written, Death is swallowed up in victory. O death, where is thy sting? O grave, where is thy victory? The sting of death is sin; and the strength of sin is the law. But thanks be to God, which giveth us the victory through our Lord Jesus Christ. Therefore, my beloved brethren, be ye stedfast, unmoveable, always abounding in the work of the Lord, forasmuch as ye know that your labour is not in vain in the Lord."
56. 2 Corinthians 1:3-4 (KJV), "Blessed be God, even the Father of our Lord Jesus Christ, the Father of mercies, and the God of all comfort; Who comforteth us in all our tribulation, that we may be able to comfort them which are in any trouble, by the comfort wherewith we ourselves are comforted of God."

CAREGIVING

57. 2 Corinthians 4:1 (KJV), "Therefore seeing we have this ministry, as we have received mercy, we faint not;"
58. 2 Corinthians 4:2 (KJV), "But have renounced the hidden things of dishonesty, not walking in craftiness, nor handling the word of God deceitfully; but by manifestation of the truth commending ourselves to every man's conscience in the sight of God."
59. 2 Corinthians 4:5(KJV), "For we preach not ourselves, but Christ Jesus the Lord; and ourselves your servants for Jesus' sake."
60. 2 Corinthians 4:7 (KJV), "But we have this treasure in earthen vessels, that the excellency of the power may be of God, and not of us."
61. 2 Corinthians 4:8-9 (KJV), "We are troubled on every side, yet not distressed; we are perplexed, but not in despair; Persecuted, but not forsaken; cast down, but not destroyed;"
62. 2 Corinthians 4:15 (KJV), "For all things are for your sakes, that the abundant grace might through the thanksgiving of many redound to the glory of God."
63. 2 Corinthians 4:16 (KJV), "For which cause we faint not; but though our outward man perish, yet the inward man is renewed day by day."
64. 2 Corinthians 4:16-18 (KJV), "For which cause we faint not; but though our outward man perish, yet the inward man is renewed day by day. For our light affliction, which is but for a moment, worketh for us a far more exceeding and eternal weight of glory; While we look not at the things which are seen, but at the things which are not seen: for the things which are seen are temporal; but the things which are not seen are eternal."
65. 2 Corinthians 4:17-18 (KJV), "For our light affliction, which is but for a moment, worketh for us a far more exceeding and eternal weight of glory; While we look not at the things which are seen, but at the things which are not seen: for the things

which are seen are temporal; but the things which are not seen are eternal."
66. Galatians 5:5 (KJV), "For we through the Spirit wait for the hope of righteousness by faith."
67. Galatians 6:8 (KJV), "For he that soweth to his flesh shall of the flesh reap corruption; but he that soweth to the Spirit shall of the Spirit reap life everlasting."
68. Philippians 1:6 (KJV), "Being confident of this very thing, that he which hath begun a good work in you will perform it until the day of Jesus Christ:"
69. Philippians 3:13-14 (KJV), "Brethren, I count not myself to have apprehended: but this one thing I do, forgetting those things which are behind, and reaching forth unto those things which are before, I press toward the mark for the prize of the high calling of God in Christ Jesus."
70. Colossians 1:27 (KJV), "To whom God would make known what is the riches of the glory of this mystery among the Gentiles; which is Christ in you, the hope of glory:"
71. Colossians 3:1-2 (KJV), "If ye then be risen with Christ, seek those things which are above, where Christ sitteth on the right hand of God. Set your affection on things above, not on things on the earth."
72. 1 Thessalonians 5:18 (KJV), "In everything give thanks: for this is the will of God in Christ Jesus concerning you."
73. Titus 2:13 (KJV), "Looking for that blessed hope, and the glorious appearing of the great God and our Saviour Jesus Christ;"
74. Hebrews 9:28 (KJV) "So Christ was once offered to bear the sins of many; and unto them that look for him shall he appear the second time without sin unto salvation."
75. Hebrew 11:11 (KJV), "Through faith also Sara herself received strength to conceive seed, and was delivered of a child when she was past age, because she judged him faithful who had promised."

CAREGIVING

76. Hebrews 13:6 (KJV), "So that we may boldly say, The Lord is my helper, and I will not fear what man shall do unto me."
77. James 1:5 (KJV) reminds us, "If any of you lack wisdom, let him ask of God, that giveth to all men liberally, and upbraideth not; and it shall be given him."
78. James 5:7-8 (KJV), "Be patient therefore, brethren, unto the coming of the Lord. Behold, the husbandman waiteth for the precious fruit of the earth, and hath long patience for it, until he receive the early and latter rain. Be ye also patient; stablish your hearts: for the coming of the Lord draweth nigh."
79. 1 Peter 5:10 (KJV), "But the God of all grace, who hath called us unto his eternal glory by Christ Jesus, after that ye have suffered a while, make you perfect, stablish, strengthen, settle you."
80. 3 John 1:2 (KJV), "Beloved, I wish above all things that thou mayest prosper and be in health, even as thy soul prospereth."
81. Revelation 6:9-11 (KJV), "And when he had opened the fifth seal, I saw under the altar the souls of them that were slain for the word of God, and for the testimony which they held: And they cried with a loud voice, saying, How long, O Lord, holy and true, dost thou not judge and avenge our blood on them that dwell on the earth? And white robes were given unto every one of them; and it was said unto them, that they should rest yet for a little season, until their fellow servants also and their brethren, that should be killed as they were, should be fulfilled."

APPENDIX F

HOW TO ACCEPT GOD'S HOPE

F.1 MY STORY

My Story

Being a good person doesn't get you to heaven. Being saved or born-again does. Here's my story of how I accepted Jesus Christ and became a Christian.

On July 11, 1977, my life changed. If you look up that date in history, you will find nothing historically significant happened on that Sunday. It was a remarkable day for me. Sunday, July 11, 1977, was the watershed event in my life.

. . .

While attending First Baptist Church of Lakewood in Tacoma, Washington, I noticed a group of men that seemed to have what I was missing. I attended a Bible study with them.

Here I found that God has given us an essential manual for life. The manual is the Bible. God has the answers to the problems and emptiness we may face. I found out I was here for a purpose, and not by accident. I learned Jesus loves me and desires to have a personal relationship with me. However, sin separated me from Him.

F.2 I REALIZED I HAD A SIN PROBLEM

The Bible says in Romans 3:23 (KJV), "For all have sinned and fall short of the glory of God."

But no one is perfect! We have all sinned and therefore cannot save ourselves by just living a good life.

Why not?

The Bible says in Romans 6:23 (KJV), "For the wages of sin is death; but the gift of God is eternal life through Jesus Christ our Lord."

F.3 I LEARNED GOD GIVES US A PROMISE

The Bible says in John 3:16 (KJV), "For God so loved the world, that he gave his only begotten Son, that whosoever believeth in him shall not perish, but have everlasting life."

CAREGIVING

F.4 I LEARNED THAT GOD MADE A PROVISION FOR ME

The Bible says in Romans 10:9-10, 13 (KJV), "That if thou shalt confess with thy mouth the Lord Jesus, and shalt believe in thine heart that God hath raised him from the dead, thou shalt be saved. For with the heart man believeth unto righteousness; and with the mouth confession is made unto salvation. For whosoever shall call upon the name of the Lord shall be saved."

F.5 I PRAYED TO ACCEPT THE GIFT OF ETERNAL LIFE THROUGH JESUS

I prayed, "Jesus, I know that I am a sinner. I believe that You died for my sins and rose from the grave so that I might have eternal life in Heaven with You. I willingly repent of my sins and ask you to come into my heart and life. Take control of my words, thoughts, and actions. I place all of my trust in You for my salvation. I accept You as my Lord and Savior, and this free gift of eternal life. Amen."

Since then my life has not been perfect. It's been far from it. I've messed up from time to time, sometimes failing miserably in my decisions and choices. However, I have had direction and purpose in my life. I know where I am headed. I have the Bible to give me the principles for daily living. I am never alone. I have had real peace for the last 40 plus years.

How about you? Have you ever been saved?

F.6 YOU CAN DO LIKE I DID

Romans 10:9-10, 13 tells us, "That if thou shalt confess with thy mouth the Lord Jesus, and shalt believe in thine heart that God hath raised him from the dead, thou shalt be saved. For with the heart man believeth unto righteousness, and with the mouth confession is made unto salvation. ... For whosoever shall call upon the name of the Lord shall be saved."

Why Not Pray This Simple Prayer and Accept Jesus Christ Today?

ABOUT THE AUTHOR

Jimmie Aaron Kepler is a full-time nonfiction writer, novelist, poet, and award-winning short story writer.

Jimmie earned a Bachelor of Arts in History with minors in English and Military Science from The University of Texas at Arlington, Master of Religious Education and Master of Arts degrees from Southwestern Baptist Theological Seminary, and the Doctor of Education degree from Pacific Western University.

A former captain in the US Army officer, Jimmie also has worked as a religious educator, corporate trainer, and information technology software and systems engineer. He lives in North Texas with his cat, Lacey. He is a widower with three grown children and one grandchild.

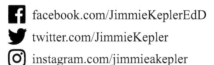

HOW TO CONTACT JIMMIE

You can sign up for the email list at:
jimmiekepler.com

Made in the USA
Las Vegas, NV
06 May 2021